INTERMITTENT FASTING FOR WOMEN OVER 60

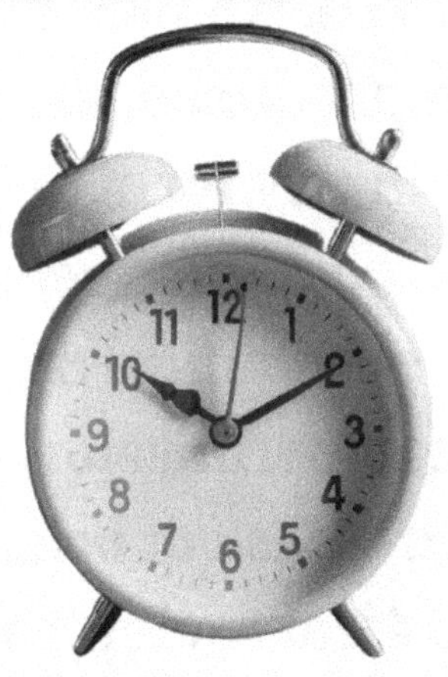

THE COMPLETE STEP-BY-STEP GUIDE TO LOSE WEIGHT, IMPROVE METABOLISM AND REDUCE AGING

HENDERSON STELLA

TABLE OF CONTENT

1. Introduction to Intermittent Fasting.............................7
- Understanding Intermittent Fasting
- Benefits for Women Over 60
- Preparing Your Body and Mind

2. The Science of Fasting and Aging..........................15
- How Fasting Affects Metabolism
- Fasting and Longevity
- Hormonal Balance and Fasting

3. Creating Your Fasting Plan.................................21
- Assessing Your Health and Lifestyle
- Setting Realistic Goals
- Personalizing Your Fasting Schedule

4. Nutrition Fundamentals......................................27
- Macronutrients and Micronutrients
- Hydration and Intermittent Fasting
- Supplements and Fasting

5. Fasting Safely and Effectively...............................33
- Common Myths and Misconceptions
- Managing Hunger and Cravings
- Fasting and Physical Activity

6. Meal Planning and Preparation............................39
- Kitchen Essentials for Healthy Cooking
- Batch Cooking and Food Storage
- Mindful Eating Practices

7. Breakfast Recipes...47
- Avocado and Egg Toast
- Greek Yogurt with Berries and Nuts
- Oatmeal with Almond Butter and Banana
- Spinach and Feta Omelette
- Chia Seed Pudding
- Smoked Salmon and Cream Cheese Wrap
- Cottage Cheese with Pineapple
- Veggie Breakfast Scramble
- Protein Smoothie
- Almond Flour Pancakes

8. Lunch Recipes...57
- Mediterranean Quinoa Salad
- Grilled Chicken Avocado Wrap
- Lentils Soup
- Tuna Salad Stuffed Bell Peppers
- Spinach and Mushroom Frittata
- Asian Chicken Salad
- Quiche with Sweet Potato Crust
- Veggie Hummus Wrap
- Tomato Basil Soup
- Roasted Vegetable and Quinoa Bowl

9. Dinner Recipes...67
- Baked Salmon with Asparagus
- Stir-Fried Tofu and Broccoli
- Zucchini Noodles with Pesto
- Cauliflower Fried Rice
- Grilled Vegetable Skewers

- Lemon Herb Chicken
- Beef and Broccoli Stir-Fry
- Stuffed Bell Peppers
- Eggplant Parmesan
- Shrimp and Arugula Salad

10. Overcoming Challenges..............................77
- Dealing with Social Situations
- Emotional Eating and Fasting
- Adjusting Your Plan as You Age

Conclusion 83
21 Days Meal Plan 84

1

INTRODUCTION TO INTERMITTENT FASTING

UNDERSTANDING INTERMITTENT FASTING

A variety of diets that alternate between periods of fasting and non-fasting for a predetermined amount of time are referred to as intermittent fasting (IF). It's not just a diet; rather, it's a style of eating that involves planning your meals to maximise their nutritional value. When you eat, rather than what you consume, is altered by IF.

Intermittent fasting is a very old concept nearly as old as human history. Fasting has historically been a feature of human behaviour, either as a result of a lack of resources or as a spiritual practice. It has been more popular in recent years as a way to get healthier and lose weight. Its appeal stems from the fact that, in comparison to other diet regimens, it is both effective and rather straightforward to adhere to.

There are many advantages to intermittent fasting for women over 60. It is well known to aid in weight loss, enhance metabolic health, and perhaps most importantly—possibly lengthen life. Intermittent fasting has been demonstrated in studies to increase insulin sensitivity and lower blood sugar, two important aspects of controlling and preventing diabetes. Furthermore, IF can lessen inflammation, which is a major cause of many common illnesses.

HOW DOES INTERMITTENT FASTING WORK?

The way intermittent fasting works is by delaying the point at which your body starts burning fat after burning through the calories from your most recent meal. It is a powerful technique to control how much energy your body uses and enhance your general well-being. There are a number of approaches to intermittent fasting, such as the eat-stop-eat approach, the 16/8 method, and the 5:2 diet. There are restrictions on what can be eaten and when for each approach.

THE 16/8 METHOD

The 16/8 approach calls for limiting your daily eating window to 8–10 hours and fasting for 14–16 hours every day. You can fit two, three, or more meals inside the allotted time for dining. Martin Berkhan, a fitness specialist, popularised the Leangains programme, another name for this approach.

THE 5:2 DIET

The 5:2 diet, sometimes referred to as The Fast Diet, calls for eating regularly five days a week and capping calories at 500–600 on the other two. Michael Mosley, a British journalist, popularised this diet.

EAT-STOP-EAT

Eat-Stop-Eat calls for one or two 24-hour fasts every week. Fitness guru Brad Pilon popularised this technique, which has gained a lot of traction over the years.

The most effective intermittent fasting technique varies from person to person. While selecting a fasting technique, factors like lifestyle, health objectives, and personal preferences should be taken into account. Before beginning any new diet, it's crucial to speak with a healthcare professional, particularly for women over 60 who may need to address certain health issues.

Starting an intermittent fasting journey might be difficult, but it can also be beneficial if you have the correct attitude and are ready. Begin by determining which approach best suits your needs and schedule your eating and fasting times. To make sure your body gets the nutrition it needs, it's critical to eat a diet rich in nutritious, nutrient-dense foods within your designated meal windows.

A great strategy for enhancing longevity and health is intermittent fasting, particularly for women over 60.

You can choose the intermittent fasting strategy that works best for you by being aware of the fundamentals of the practice and the various approaches that are out there. Recall that the purpose of intermittent fasting is to enhance general health and wellbeing rather than only reduce weight.

This overview of intermittent fasting lays the groundwork for the remainder of the book, which delves deeper into every facet of this eating style and equips you with the skills and information required to effectively incorporate intermittent fasting into your daily routine.

BENEFIT FOR WOMEN OVER 60

The possible health benefits of intermittent fasting (IF) have drawn attention, especially for women over the age of sixty. By adopting IF into their lifestyle, this population can see notable gains in a number of health indicators and quality of life. Let's investigate the advantages that IF has to offer.

- Enhanced Metabolic Well-being

The improvement in metabolic health is one of the main advantages of IF for women over 60. Our metabolism naturally slows down as we get older, which can result in weight gain and related health problems. By improving the body's sensitivity to insulin, IF can speed up metabolism, improve blood sugar regulation, and lower the risk of type 2 diabetes.

- Control of Weight

For many women over 60, weight control is a regular worry. Because IF makes eating easier and can naturally lower calorie consumption, it can be a helpful technique for weight management. Additionally, the fasting intervals stimulate the body to use fat that has been stored as fuel, which may result in weight loss.

- Improved Mental Performance

According to recently published research, IF may provide neuroprotective benefits.

This is especially advantageous for women over 60 who may be worried about cognitive deterioration. Brain-derived neurotrophic factor (BDNF), a protein involved in memory, learning, and the development of new neurons, can be produced in greater quantities during fasting.

• Reduced Sensitivity to Injury

Numerous age-related illnesses are associated with chronic inflammation. By lowering inflammation levels in the body, IF may help minimise the chance of developing long-term illnesses like Alzheimer's, arthritis, and heart disease.

• Maximum Autophagy

The body uses autophagy to eliminate damaged cells and make room for the regeneration of healthy, new ones. IF has the ability to speed up autophagy, which is advantageous for cellular upkeep and repair. In order to promote longevity and lessen the consequences of ageing, this process is essential.

• Healthy Heart

For women over 60, cardiovascular health is a big concern. It has been demonstrated that IF improves a number of cardiovascular risk variables, such as triglycerides, cholesterol, and blood pressure.

• Synaptic Balance

Although hormonal changes are a normal aspect of ageing, they can potentially have negative health effects. Hormones like insulin and human growth hormone (HGH) can be balanced with the use of IF, and this can benefit bone health, muscle strength, and general vigour.

• Enhanced Digestive Wellness

Frequent fasting intervals can provide the digestive system with a much-needed respite, facilitating improved nutrition absorption and digestion after meals. This may result in less digestive problems and better gut health.

- Improved Physical Capabilities

Contrary to popular belief, IF can improve physical performance. Fasting can help women over 60 maintain or even increase their strength and endurance since it can enhance muscular efficiency and recovery when done under the right supervision.

- Psychological Wellness

Emotional well-being can benefit from IF as well. For women over 60, the structure and discipline of IF can foster a sense of control and accomplishment. Furthermore, any gains in physical health may result in elevated mood and self-worth.

Women over 60 can benefit from intermittent fasting in several ways that improve their physical and emotional well-being. Women can make wise judgements concerning IF integration by being aware of these advantages. To ensure that readers may take advantage of these advantages and still enjoy tasty and nourishing meals, the next chapters will offer comprehensive instructions on how to practise IF safely and successfully.

PREPARATION YOUR BODY AND MIND

Starting an intermittent fasting (IF) journey is a holistic method that entails mentally and physically preparing yourself. It's not simply about changing your meal pattern. This preparation is essential for women over 60 to guarantee a safe and successful fasting experience. This section will walk you through the process of getting ready for IF, emphasising mental toughness, emotional support, and physical preparedness.

It is vital to evaluate your physical health before beginning IF. Speak with a healthcare professional about any current ailments and prescription drugs. This stage helps customise the fasting strategy to meet your needs and guarantees that IF is suitable for you.

Adjust your diet gradually to ease yourself into IF. Start by consuming more whole foods, such as fruits, vegetables, lean meats, and healthy fats, and fewer processed meals. This change amplifies the benefits of fasting and gets your body ready for it.

Acquire the ability to distinguish between actual hunger and habitual eating. You may feel hungry at times when you're used to eating during the early phases of IF. Understanding these cues enables you to better control your hunger during fasting times.
It's crucial to stay hydrated, particularly during the times when you fast. Hydration and hunger control can be achieved with the aid of water, herbal teas, and other non-caloric liquids.

As vital as physical preparedness is mental preparation. IF necessitates self-control and a change in perspective about food and meals.
Establish measurable objectives for your IF journey. Whether your goal is more energy, better health markers, or weight loss, setting precise goals helps you stay motivated and focused.

It gives you the ability to make wise selections if you know how IF works and its advantages. To learn more and get support, read up about IF, go to workshops, or participate in internet forums.

Go into IF with an optimistic attitude. Accept the adjustments as a component of a better way of life as opposed to a rigorous diet. To be upbeat, acknowledge and appreciate your little accomplishments along the road.

Having a network of support can make IF much more enjoyable. Tell loved ones or friends about your plans so they can support you.

Think about getting involved in an online or local IF community. Making connections with people who are on similar paths fosters a sense of camaraderie and offers a forum for exchanging advice and experiences.

Stress can obstruct your IF objectives. Take part in stress-relieving exercises, yoga, meditation, or mild physical activity. These exercises enhance your general wellbeing in addition to lowering tension.

As you adjust to IF, practise self-compassion and patience. Experiences of highs and lows are common. Pay attention to your body and modify your fasting schedule as necessary.

A successful intermittent fasting (IF) journey begins with preparing your body and mind in a methodical way. Through careful preparation of your body, development of your mental toughness, and seeking out emotional support, you may face the challenges of IF with poise and assurance. Building on this preparation, the upcoming chapters will walk you through the practical aspects of IF and provide you the tools you need to incorporate it easily into your daily life.

2

THE SCIENCE OF FASTING AND AGING

HOW FASTING AFFECTS METABOLISM

The biochemical processes that a living thing goes through to stay alive are referred to as metabolism. It consists of two primary parts: anabolism, which is the synthesis of all the substances required by the cells, and catabolism, which is the breakdown of molecules to obtain energy.

Our metabolism slows down as we become older for a variety of reasons, including hormonal shifts, loss of muscle mass, and reduced physical activity. This can make it difficult for women over 60 to maintain a healthy weight and level of energy.

There are various ways that intermittent fasting might affect metabolism. When a person fasts, their body uses up all of its sugar reserves and enters a state known as ketosis, when they burn fat for energy. This change helps the body burn fat more quickly and increases metabolic flexibility, which makes it easier for the body to transition between fuel sources.

The increase in insulin sensitivity that results with IF is one of its main metabolic advantages. Insulin is released during feeding to facilitate the uptake of glucose by cells from the circulation. Frequent eating can eventually cause insulin resistance, a disease in which cells lose their ability to respond to insulin. By resetting this sensitivity, IF lowers the chance of developing type 2 diabetes.

Research has demonstrated that IF can raise the body's resting metabolic rate (RMR), or the amount of calories burned while at rest. Even when not actively exercising, a higher RMR indicates that the body is using energy more efficiently.

These include more growth hormone release, which maintains muscular mass and function, and elevated norepinephrine levels, which can speed up metabolism.

Fasting stimulates autophagy, the body's cellular "cleanup" mechanism. By getting rid of broken parts that can slow down metabolic processes, this not only promotes cellular health but also a healthy metabolism.

Women over 60 may require some time to adjust to IF. It's crucial to begin cautiously and pay attention to your body's signals. The body can adapt by gradually lengthening fasting times without putting too much strain on it.

FASTING AND LONGEVITY

The progressive deterioration of biological processes and the body's capacity to adjust to metabolic stress are hallmarks of ageing, which is an inevitable aspect of life. Cellular alterations such as DNA damage, telomere shortening, and diminished cellular repair systems are involved.

Cellular health has been demonstrated to be significantly impacted by intermittent fasting. IF triggers metabolic stress periods, which open up cellular pathways essential for cellular renewal and repair. The sirtuin family of proteins, which is linked to lifespan and stress resistance, is one of these pathways.
The body uses autophagy, a crucial mechanism during fasting, to eliminate damaged cells so that healthy, new ones can grow in their place. Improved health outcomes and a longer lifespan are linked to enhanced autophagy.

Age-related illnesses like cardiovascular disease, neurological disorders, and several forms of cancer can be lowered by IF. By lowering inflammation and enhancing metabolic health, IF supports the body's resistance to various illnesses

The key to IF's longevity benefits is the idea of hormesis, which describes the positive consequences of mild stress. The body experiences a slight stress during a fast, which can fortify cellular defences and lengthen life.

Growth hormone (GH) is a major factor in the ageing process. While GH secretion generally decreases with age, fasting can enhance it, which benefits bone density, muscle mass, and general vigour.

Ageing has been associated with Insulin-like Growth Factor (IGF-1), a hormone that resembles insulin. Reduced IGF-1 levels, which arise during fasting, are linked to longer lifespans in a variety of species.

IF may also have an effect on the mental effects of ageing. Successful adherence to an IF regimen can lead to discipline and empowerment, which can enhance mental health and promote a more optimistic view of ageing.Research on the connection between longevity and intermittent fasting is quite promising, particularly for women over the age of sixty. Women can decrease their risk of age-related disorders and stimulate biological pathways that support healthy ageing by participating in IF. The parts that follow will go into greater detail about fasting and hormone balance, giving women a thorough guidance to utilising the anti-aging benefits of intermittent fasting.

HORMONAL BALANCE AND FASTING

After wrapping up the second chapter of "Intermittent Fasting for Women Over 60," we'll concentrate on how hormonal balance plays a crucial part in ageing and how intermittent fasting (IF) might help maintain it.

Hormones are chemical messengers that are essential for controlling metabolism, development, and reproduction, among other body processes. Hormonal changes throughout ageing can cause a variety of age-related alterations and health problems in women.

One of the main female sex hormones, oestrogen, dramatically drops during and after menopause, which may result in mood changes, weight gain, and an increased risk of osteoporosis. By supporting bone health and encouraging a healthy body composition, IF can help lessen these impacts.

One hormone that controls blood glucose levels is insulin. Age-related decreases in insulin sensitivity can result in elevated blood sugar levels and a higher chance of type 2 diabetes. It has been demonstrated that IF increases insulin sensitivity, which helps with glucose management.

The stress hormone cortisol can be harmful if levels are persistently high, as they are during extended periods of stress. Cortisol regulation with IF can result in a more balanced stress response and enhanced general wellbeing.

It takes thyroid hormones to keep the metabolic rate constant. Differenciates in thyroid function may result in metabolic problems. By regulating hormone levels and improving metabolic processes, IF can help maintain the health of the thyroid.

The health of bones and muscles is significantly influenced by HGH. Fasting can enhance the synthesis of human growth hormone (HGH), which counteracts some of the effects of ageing by supporting tissue repair and maintenance as well as helping to maintain lean muscle mass.

Ghrelin and leptin control hunger and fullness. By balancing these hormones, IF might lessen excessive hunger cues and encourage more restrained eating habits.

The body's capacity to break down fats is improved by adiponectin, which is secreted by fat cells. Adiponectin levels can be raised by IF, which enhances fat metabolism and helps with weight management.

Ageing can have an impact on melatonin synthesis, which controls sleep patterns. By affecting melatonin synthesis, IF may enhance the quality of sleep, resulting in improved relaxation and recuperation.

The foundation of good health is hormonal balance, particularly for women over 60. A novel strategy for reestablishing this equilibrium is intermittent fasting, which may also have a favourable effect on other hormonal pathways. Women can enhance their health, vigour, and longevity by comprehending and utilising the hormonal advantages of intermittent fasting.

3

CREATING YOUR FASTING PLAN

ACCESSING YOUR HEALTH AND LIFESTYLE

It is imperative that you take a close look at your present state of health and way of living. This first step is essential to ensure a safe and successful fasting experience and customising the intermittent fasting (IF) approach to your unique needs.

Prior to putting IF into practice, it's critical to comprehend your beginning point. This entails closely examining your eating patterns, exercise routine, and any underlying medical concerns that may have an impact on your capacity to fast.

A thorough medical examination performed by a qualified healthcare provider might reveal important information about your health. A review of your medical history, current medications, and any possible dangers related to fasting should all be included in this. Blood tests can also be used to evaluate your baseline metabolic health, which includes cholesterol and blood sugar levels.

How you adjust to IF depends a lot on your lifestyle. Think about your dietary habits, social obligations, and daily schedule. Do you like to eat larger meals later in the day, or are you an early riser who loves breakfast? Knowing these behaviours will enable you to select an IF regimen that fits your way of life.

When designing an IF regimen, women over 60 have certain dietary demands that need to be taken into account. Protein, calcium, and vitamin D are especially crucial for maintaining healthy bones and muscles. To satisfy these demands, make sure that your diet consists of a range of nutrient-dense foods.

21

Frequent exercise can support your IF plan and is a crucial part of general wellness. Evaluate your present level of activity and think about ways to increase your daily physical activity, such as regular walks or gardening, or more scheduled exercise.

For your IF journey, establish attainable and reasonable goals based on your assessment of your health and lifestyle. These objectives should provide your fasting strategy a defined direction and be time-bound, measurable, and explicit.

You can start tailoring your fasting schedule with the data you obtained from your examination. Select a fasting technique that works for your daily schedule, nutritional requirements, and state of health. Keep in mind that IF is adaptable, therefore it's critical to discover a rhythm that suits your needs.

To ensure that your IF experience is successful, you must first evaluate your lifestyle and health. By taking the time to comprehend your particular circumstances, you can design a customised fasting schedule that complements your wellness objectives and works well with your daily schedule.

SETTING REALISTIC GOALS

Decide why you want to start IF first. Is it to boost your general well-being, enhance your metabolic health, or help you lose weight? Setting relevant and inspiring goals is made easier when you are aware of your own motives.

SMART Objective Establishment
Goals ought to be Specific, Measurable, Achievable, Relevant and Time Bound (SMART). A SMART goal may be, for example, "to lose 10 pounds in 3 months by practicing the 16/8 intermittent fasting method and engaging in 30 minutes of moderate exercise daily," as opposed to just wanting to "lose weight."

- Specific

Give your objectives as much detail as you can. Rather than settling for a general objective such as "eat healthier," define what healthy eating means to you. It might say "incorporate at least two servings of vegetables into my meals daily."

- Measurable Goals

Make sure your objectives can be measured. Establish what improving your metabolic health means if that is your objective. It might "reduce my fasting blood glucose levels to under 100 mg/dL."

- Achievable Goals

Make sure your goals are reachable and reasonable. Think about your lifestyle, responsibilities, and state of health right now. A goal like "run a marathon" can be too ambitious if you're just starting out with exercise. Rather, strive to "walk 10,000 steps a day."

- Realistic goals

Your long-term health aims and your life should be in line with your ambitions. Your objective can be to "perform weight-bearing exercises three times a week" if increasing bone density is a priority.

- Time Bound

Set a deadline for your objectives. This can encourage you to keep moving forward by fostering a sense of urgency. over instance, "increase my water intake to 64 ounces a day for the next month."

Your objectives could change as you work with IF more. Review and modify your goals frequently to take into account your present circumstances. It's possible for something difficult to become less difficult, and you may adjust your goals to keep pushing and motivating yourself.

Part of your IF experience is fundamentally setting reasonable goals. You may clearly outline your fasting regimen by taking the time to set SMART goals. Maintaining focus and drive while navigating the path to increased health and vitality requires this clarity and direction.

PERSONALIZING YOUR FASTING SCHEDULE

Circadian rhythms are the unique natural cycles and rhythms that each person's body has. You can choose the ideal times to eat and fast by keeping an eye on these. For example, you may prefer a fasting schedule that permits an earlier dinner if you are an early riser.

There are various IF techniques, each with a unique set of rules. The well-liked 16/8 regimen, which calls for a 16-hour fast followed by an 8-hour interval for eating, could be a good place to start. If this doesn't work for your lifestyle, though, you could try alternate-day fasting or the 5:2 technique.

When organising your fasting schedule, take into account your daily schedule. If you frequently have dinner parties for friends, it can be better to have a later eating window. On the other hand, if you like having breakfast meetings, you might benefit from an earlier dining window.

Start with a trial period to discover how your selected timetable works within your daily routine. As you get more insight into what suits you best, it's acceptable to modify your eating and fasting times. Sustaining an IF practice over the long run requires flexibility.

Keep a close eye on how fasting affects your body. Feeling alert and invigorated is a positive indicator. But if you feel lethargic or have other unpleasant symptoms, it might be time to reevaluate your schedule.

Pay attention to the timing of your nutrients when you consume. Benefits of IF can be increased by consuming the appropriate foods at the appropriate times. For instance, consuming protein post-exercise can help with muscle repair, but consuming carbohydrates earlier in the day can provide more energy.

You shouldn't be emotionally or socially isolated by IF. Arrange your fasting period to coincide with significant family get-togethers and social events. Making IF a harmonious aspect of your life rather than a burdensome restriction is the aim.

Finding the ideal balance that suits your needs is the first step in customising your fasting plan. You can design an IF regimen that complements your health objectives and blends in with your regular routine by taking into account your body's natural rhythms, lifestyle, and nutritional requirements.

4

NUTRITION FUNDAMENTAL

MACRONUTRIENTS AND MICRONUTRIENTS

The Part Macronutrients Plays
The larger-quantity nutrients carbohydrates, proteins, and fats that provide us energy are known as macronutrients. Everybody has a distinct role to play in preserving health, particularly for women over 60.

Carbohydrates: The main energy source for the body. Whole grains and other complex carbs are better for you than simple sugars since they have fibre to help with digestion and provide long-lasting energy.

Proteins: Vital for tissue repair and muscle maintenance, proteins play a bigger role in preventing sarcopenia, the age-related loss of muscle mass, as we age.

Fats: Good fats, especially omega-3 fatty acids, lower inflammation and promote mental wellness. You should incorporate foods like almonds, avocados, and olive oil in your diet.

Knowing About Micronutrients
Although micronutrients, such as vitamins and minerals, are needed in lesser quantities, they are essential for maintaining general health and preventing deficits.

Vitamins: Antioxidants including vitamins C and E assist prevent oxidative stress, while vitamins D, B12, and calcium are essential for healthy bones.

Minerals: Iron, magnesium, and potassium are among the minerals that are important for heart health, muscle function, and the synthesis of energy.

Achieving Nutrient Balance with IF

Making ensuring your eating windows include the right ratio of macro and micronutrients to suit your body's demands is crucial when following an IF regimen. When meals are limited to specific times, this can be difficult, but it is possible with careful preparation.

Pay attention to foods that are high in nutrients compared to their calorie content, or those that are nutrient-dense. Good options include foods like beans, berries, leafy greens, and lean meats.

To achieve your micronutrient demands, supplements could be required in some circumstances, particularly if your dietary consumption is restricted. It is advisable to speak with a healthcare professional first before beginning any supplementation, though.

Water is necessary for life even though it isn't a nutrient and is important for nutrient absorption. Make sure you stay hydrated all day, especially if you're fasting.

The fundamental components of a nutritious diet are macronutrients and micronutrients. Knowing and including these nutrients in your diet is essential for women over 60 who follow intermittent fasting (IF) in order to sustain their energy levels, support their bodies, and improve their general health.

HYDRATION AND INTERMITTENT FASTING

For people's health and wellbeing, especially for women over 60 who are intermittent fasting (IF), hydration is essential. The necessity of staying properly hydrated and how it relates to IF procedures will be covered in detail in this portion of the book.

The Body's Requirement of Water

Life need water. It facilitates metabolic reactions, aids in regulating body temperature, facilitates digestion, and is essential for the transportation of nutrients and the removal of waste. Maintaining these processes requires adequate hydration, particularly during fasting periods when food intake is restricted.

Fasting and Hydration

You are not allowed to consume any calories during periods of fasting, including those from hydration-containing liquids. It's crucial to pay attention to how much water you consume during these periods. Headaches, exhaustion, and lightheadedness brought on by dehydration might be misinterpreted as signs of hunger or discomfort from fasting.

Amount of Water Required?

The amount of water required might change depending on a person's weight, age, activity level, and climate. Aiming for at least 8 to 10 cups (64 to 80 ounces) of water per day is a general recommendation, although this may need to be modified for individual needs.

Dehydration Signs

It is critical to recognise the symptoms of dehydration. Dry lips, reduced urination, dark yellow urine, dry skin, and dizziness are a few of them. Up your water intake if you encounter these symptoms.

Including Foods That Are Hydrating
Consuming foods that are high in water content will help you meet your daily fluid needs in addition to drinking water. Foods with a high water content that you can include in your eating windows include cucumbers, tomatoes, oranges, and melons.

Electrolyte Balance
Your body may lose electrolytes through urine when you fast, especially if you do so for extended periods of time. Maintaining the proper balance of electrolytes like magnesium, potassium, and sodium is crucial. When you eat, think about eating foods high in electrolytes or adding a bit of salt to your drink.

IF Hydration Techniques
The objective is to create a hydration plan that complements your intermittent fasting regimen. Here are some things you could find useful: - Have a big glass of water to start your day.
- Carry a water bottle with you during the day so you may take frequent sips.
- Have a glass of water both before and after the end of your fasting period.

It's important to remember to stay hydrated when doing IF. It's an easy yet powerful approach to guarantee a healthy and productive fasting experience. You can support your body's demands, prevent the dangers of dehydration, and increase the efficacy of your IF regimen by maintaining proper hydration.

SUPPLEMENT AND FASTING

It is worthwhile to investigate supplements because this age group may have unique nutritional needs that are not usually satisfied by diet alone.

Our bodies becoming less adept at absorbing nutrients from meals as we get older, and some medical disorders or prescription drugs can make this process much more difficult. By ensuring that you have all the vitamins and minerals you need to sustain your health, supplements can help close nutritional gaps in your diet.

Typical Vitamins for Women Over 60
Vitamin D: Supplementing with Vitamin D is frequently required, particularly for individuals who have limited sun exposure, as it is essential for immune system and bone health.

Calcium: Supplementing with calcium is beneficial for preserving bone density, especially for women who have gone through menopause.

Omega-3 Fatty Acids: These may not be obtained in sufficient amounts from diet alone, but they support heart and brain function.

vitamins B: Due to aging-related decreased absorption, B12, in particular, which is essential for nerve function and energy production, may need to be supplemented.

Magnesium: Supporting blood sugar regulation, blood pressure regulation, and muscle and nerve function, magnesium is involved in over 300 metabolic activities in the body.

Fasting Windows and Supplements
It's crucial to think about the timing of your supplements when implementing IF. Vitamins A, D, E, and K are among the fat-soluble vitamins that are best absorbed when taken with food. Some can be taken on an empty stomach since they are water soluble, such as vitamin C and B vitamins.

Recognise the possibility of drug and supplement interactions. Before beginning any new supplement, see a doctor, especially if you are using medication or have underlying medical issues.

Supplements are not made equally. Seek for goods that have undergone independent testing to ensure their purity and quality. In order to prevent any negative effects, it's also critical to adhere to the specified dosages.

Try to obtain your nutrition from whole foods whenever you can. Supplements should be used in addition to a balanced diet, not in place of it, especially if you have dietary restrictions or medical problems that make it difficult for you to get all the nutrients you need from food alone.

For women over 60 adopting an IF lifestyle, supplements can be helpful in ensuring that all nutritional requirements are satisfied. Without sacrificing your nutritional status, you can optimise the health benefits of intermittent fasting (IF) by strategically choosing and scheduling your supplements.

5

FASTING SAFELY AND EFFECTIVELY

COMMON MYTHS AND MISCONCEPTIONS

The idea that fasting equates to famine is among the most widely held misconceptions. On the other hand, malnutrition, or starving, results from the body being denied vital nutrients for a prolonged length of time. In contrast, intermittent fasting (IF) is a methodical and regulated way to plan eating and fasting windows that enable the body to burn fat stores as fuel while still getting enough nutrients.

The loss of muscle during fasting is another issue. Although the body can metabolise protein for energy, this is not the main way that the body gets fuel when fasting. The body consumes its reserves of glycogen before switching to fat. Furthermore, IF can raise growth hormone levels, which contribute to the preservation of muscle mass.

While evidence indicates that short-term fasting can actually enhance metabolic rate by promoting norepinephrine release, which boosts metabolism, many people still assume that fasting slows down metabolism. A prolonged reduction in calories without fasting may cause a decrease in metabolism.

Some believe that older folks should not use IF. But when implemented properly, IF can provide seniors with a host of health advantages, such as better metabolic health, elevated insulin sensitivity, and improved cognitive performance. Before beginning any new diet, it's crucial to speak with a healthcare professional, especially for those who already have medical issues

Even though IF doesn't specify what you consume, it's still critical to select wholesome foods that satisfy your body's requirements.

Eating a diet high in whole foods, lean proteins, healthy fats, and veggies will enhance general health and augment the benefits of intermittent fasting.

Many people believe that IF cannot be sustained over time. But because IF is adaptable and can be tailored to suit unique preferences and lifestyles, it's a viable option for a lot of people, including women over 60.

Anyone thinking about IF needs to know the truth behind these myths and misconceptions. For women over 60, intermittent fasting (IF) can be a safe and efficient way to enhance health and well-being with the correct information and methodology. In order to assist readers in making knowledgeable decisions regarding IF, the remainder of this chapter will continue to examine more widespread myths and offer evidence-based corrections.

MANAGING HUNGER AND CRAVINGS

First, it's critical to distinguish between cravings and hunger, which are different physiological needs for food that are frequently fueled by habits, emotions, or the urge for sensory gratification. Understanding the distinction will enable you to react correctly.

Means of Handling Hunger
Remain Hydrated: Many times, thirst is confused with hunger. Make sure you have adequate water to drink during the day.

Increase Fibre Intake: Vegetables and whole grains, which are high in fibre, might make you feel satiated for longer.

Eat Foods High in Protein: Protein helps you feel full and reduce hunger because it has a high satiety index.

Practice Mindful Eating: Take note of what you're eating, relish every bite, and pay attention to your body's fullness cues.

Overcoming Cravings

- Identify Triggers: Record urges in your journal as they happen. Finding trends will assist you in addressing the root problems.

- Find Healthy Alternatives: Fruit is a healthier choice than sugary snacks when you're craving something sweet.

- Distract Yourself: Take up a mental diversion from food, such as making a phone call or going for a walk.

- Allow for Flexibility: You can avoid overindulging later on by occasionally treating yourself to a tiny piece of what you're craving.

Emotion-Driven Food

- Cravings may be significantly influenced by emotional eating. It's critical to learn non-food coping mechanisms for emotions:
- Stress MManagement: You can handle stress without turning to food by practicing techniques like deep breathing, meditation, or yoga.

- Seek Support: Sharing your feelings with friends, family, or a support group might help you feel better and lessen the emotional need to eat.

- Make Nutritious Snacks: Keep wholesome options on hand in case you get hungry.

- Regular Meal Times: To control your hunger hormones, try to eat at regular intervals throughout your eating window.

Controlling desires and hunger is essential to a good IF experience. You may stick to your fasting schedule and not feel hungry or deprived by using these tactics. The remainder of this chapter will examine other difficulties and offer more advice on smoothly navigating the IF journey.

FASTING AND PHYSICAL ACTIVITIES

IF can benefit from physical activity. It can be beneficial:

- Increase Fat Burning: Engaging in exercise during a fast may enhance the body's capacity to burn fat for energy.

- Improve Metabolic Health: Another advantage of IF is that it can improve insulin sensitivity with consistent exercise.

- Improve Mental Clarity: Many people claim that fasting increases their mental attentiveness, which can make exercise feel more fruitful.

Exercise Types to Think About

- Low-Intensity Steady-State (LISS): Energy-spending activities that can be maintained for extended periods of time during a fast, such as walking or light cycling, are excellent choices.

- Strength Training: Maintaining muscle mass is important for women who are over 60. The ideal time to do it is just after your workout, when you can feed your muscles with protein.

- Exercises for Flexibility and Balance: Pilates and yoga can increase core strength, flexibility, and balance while requiring less energy.

- Scheduling Your Exercise
- While Fasting: If you would like to work out, try to keep your intensity low to moderate in order to accommodate your body's energy availability.

- After Eating: To guarantee you have the energy to perform and recover, schedule more strenuous activities, such as high-intensity interval training (HIIT) or weightlifting, after you've eaten.

Paying attention to your body's cues is essential. It might not be the greatest time to exercise if you feel lightheaded, weak, or exhausted. It can be beneficial to modify the duration or intensity of your workouts.

It doesn't matter when you exercise—staying hydrated is crucial. Before, during, and after physical activity, sip water to replenish fluids lost through perspiration.

Nutrition following exercise is crucial for recuperation, particularly following strength training. Arrange your fasting period such that, following your workout, you can have a high-protein, high-carb lunch.

Speak with your healthcare physician and think about working with a fitness professional to build a plan that works for you before beginning any new workout regimen, especially while fasting.

An additional component of IF that can increase its advantages is physical activity. Women over 60 can keep an active lifestyle that supports their fasting regimen and overall health goals by carefully assessing the type, timing, and intensity of exercise.

6

MEAL PLANNING AND PREPARATION

KITCHEN ESSENTIALS FOR HEALTHY COOKING

A well-stocked kitchen serves as the basis for culinary creativity, much like a canvas does for an artist. Cooking is made simpler, more effective, and more pleasurable with the correct equipment. This is particularly crucial if you have a restricted eating window and need your meals to be filling and nutritious.

Must Have Cooking Utensils
Quality Knives: Most chopping and slicing jobs may be completed with a sharp chef's knife and a paring knife.

Cutting Boards: To avoid cross-contamination, use a couple of robust cutting boards, one for produce and another for meats.

Non-Stick Cookware: Cooking with less oil is healthy when using high-quality pots and pans.

Food processor or blender: These devices work well for creating sauces, soups, and smoothies.

Measuring Cups and Spoons: Accuracy is essential in cooking, particularly when following directions or monitoring dietary consumption.

Mixing Bowls: To prepare and combine components, a collection of mixing bowls of different sizes is necessary.

Storage Containers: Meal planning and preserving the freshness of leftovers are made easier with a set of storage containers.

Sourcing Provisions
- Whole Grains: Nutritious and adaptable, quinoa, brown rice, and oats are all filled with nutrients.

- Legumes: Beans and lentils are satisfying and a great source of protein. Almonds, chia seeds, and flaxseeds are Nuts and Seeds that provide meals crunch and nutrients.

- Healthy Oils: Avocado and olive oils are heart-healthy fats that work well in dressings and cooking.

- Herbs and Spices: These enhance taste without adding calories. Stock up on a variety to add some flair to your cooking.

Basics of Refrigerators
- Fresh Produce: A diverse assortment of fruits and veggies guarantees that you're getting a whole spectrum of minerals and vitamins.

- Lean Proteins: Fish, tofu, and chicken supply the building blocks needed to maintain muscular mass.

- Dairy or Alternatives: Almond milk and Greek yoghurt are excellent providers of calcium and protein.

- Eggs: Rich in minerals and protein, eggs are adaptable and work well in a variety of recipes.

Freezer Attachments
- Frozen Fruits and Vegetables: These can be used while in-season and are just as nutrient-dense as fresh.
- Whole Grain Breads: You may keep a piece on hand at all times by freezing the slices.

- Pre-Cooked Meals: Planning ahead will help you save time and make sure you follow your IF schedule.

Structuring for Effectiveness
- Keep Essentials Within Reach: Set up your kitchen so that the most frequently used utensils and ingredients are nearby.
- Date and Label: To maintain track of freshness and contents, clearly label your storage containers, frozen meals, and seasonings.
- Sanitise as You Go: Cooking is more enjoyable in a clean kitchen since it is more welcoming.

Health Benefiting Cooking Methods
- Steaming: This method retains more nutrients in veggies than boiling.
- Grilling: Uses a grill pan indoors and adds flavour without requiring a lot of oil.
- Roasting: This hands-off cooking technique brings out the inherent sweetness in veggies.
- Sautéing: This is a quick and simple method that works well for stir-fries and other quick dishes.

A successful IF journey starts with stocking your kitchen with necessities. With the correct supplies and equipment, you can make tasty, gratifying meals that fit your fasting schedule and are also healthful. This chapter lays the groundwork for the upcoming meal plans and dishes, so you'll be ready to start this new chapter in your culinary journey.

BATCH COOKING AND FOOD STORAGE

By using these strategies, you can make meal preparation more efficient and guarantee that there are always nutritious options available when you're ready to eat.

Cooking in batches entails preparing greater amounts of food all at once and then portioning it out for use later. You may cook less often and still enjoy homemade meals with this effective and time-saving method.

Advantages of Cooking in Batch

- Dietary Consistency: Keeping prepared meals on hand facilitates adherence to IF and nutritional objectives.

- Time Management: Reduce time spent preparing meals every day by cooking once or twice a week.

- Reduced Waste: Batch cooking can help control portion sizes and cut down on food waste.

Effective Batch Cooking Techniques

- Plan Your Menu: Select dishes that are wholesome, filling, and enjoyable to prepare. Think about freezer-friendly meals.
- Smart Shop: Make a shopping list that takes into account your menu plan to make sure you have everything you need.
- Efficient Cooking: Prepare several dishes at once by using your hob, oven and other appliances.
- Control of Points: Portion cooked food according to your IF schedule and nutritional requirements.

Food Preservation Advice

- Maintaining the freshness and nutritional value of your batch-cooked meals depends on proper food storage.

- Cooling Down: To stop bacteria from growing, let food cool to room temperature before freezing or refrigerating.

- Airtight Containers: To help maintain flavour and avoid freezer burn, store food in airtight containers.

- Labelling: To maintain inventory control and guarantee appropriate rotation, label containers with the contents and the date.

- Freezing: To make defrosting and reheating meals easier, freeze them in single-serving containers.

Safe Reheating

It's important to reheat food securely when it's time to eat.
- Thawing: Use your microwave's defrost option or leave frozen meals in the fridge overnight to thaw.
- Even Heating: To guarantee that all bacteria are destroyed, reheat food until it is heated fully.
- Avoid Repeated Reheating: To preserve food safety and quality, try to reheat only what you'll eat.

Including New Components

Even though cooking in bulk is easier, adding fresh ingredients to your meals improves their flavour and nutritional value.
- Fresh Salads: To go with your warmed dish, make a fresh salad.
- Herbs and Spices: To revive flavours, add some freshly chopped herbs or a dash of spices right before serving.
- Quick Sauté: You may give your dinner a crisp, fresh texture by quickly sautéing your veggies.

For women over 60 in particular, batch cooking and efficient food storage are essential skills for navigating an intermittent fasting lifestyle. You may make sure you always have wholesome, home-cooked meals on hand, which will make it simpler to stick to your fasting schedule and dietary objectives. This can be achieved by setting aside time for meal preparation and storage.

MINDFUL EATING PRACTICE

Being totally present and involved in the eating experience is what mindful eating entails, and it can augment the advantages of intermittent fasting.

The foundation of mindful eating is the idea of mindfulness, which is an unjudging concentration on the present moment during meditation. When it comes to eating, it refers to being mindful of your body's signals of hunger and fullness as well as the flavour, texture, and aroma of your meal.

Advantages of Intentional Eating

- Improves Digestion: You can increase the rate at which nutrients are absorbed into your body by eating mindfully and chewing your food well.

- Promotes Satiety: Eating mindfully can help you avoid overindulging by assisting you in recognising when you are full.

- Increases Enjoyment: Even while eating fewer meals, you can get more satisfaction from them if you savour every bite.

- Reduces Stress: Eating thoughtfully can help you decompress and take a break from the demands of the day.

Methods for Conscious Eating

- Eat Distraction-Free: Put your phone aside, turn off the TV, and concentrate only on your food.

- Chew Thoroughly: To facilitate digestion and extend the meal experience, give each bite a few chews.

- Activate Your Senses: Take note of your food's flavours, textures, colours, and scents.
- Verify Your Physical Condition: Throughout the meal, take regular breaks to evaluate your feelings of hunger and fullness.

Establishing a Conscious Dining Space
- Set the Table: Arrange your table so that it is visually appealing and that there is little clutter.
- Portion Control: To assist control portion sizes, serve your food on smaller plates.
- Build Gratitude: Before you eat, take a moment to thank God for your food and the nourishment it offers.

Conscious Consumption and IF
You can maximise your eating windows by incorporating mindful eating into your IF schedule. It can make the shift from fasting to eating more purposeful and fulfilling and foster a closer relationship with your food.

Overcoming Obstacles
- Handling Urgency: Before starting your meal, take a few deep breaths to centre yourself if you feel hurried to finish your fasting window before it closes.
- Addressing Emotional Eating: Investigate the emotions that might be causing you to overeat, and then come up with alternate coping mechanisms.

A useful technique for changing your connection with food is mindful eating. It provides a means for women over 60 who are following IF to optimise the mental and physical health advantages of their dietary decisions. You can enhance your well-being, savour your meals to the fullest, and uphold a balanced nutritional regimen by eating mindfully.

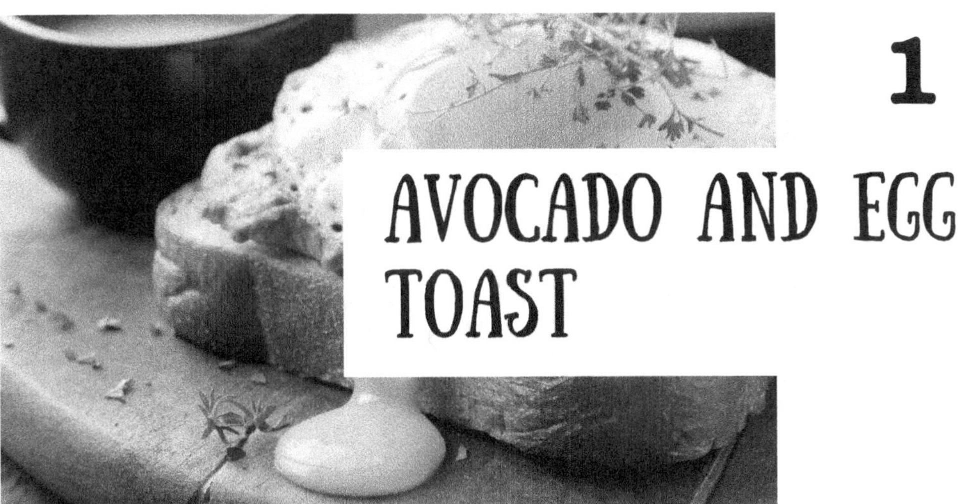

1

AVOCADO AND EGG TOAST

SERVINGS: 1

PREPPING TIME: 10 MIN

INGREDIENTS

1 slice whole-grain bread

1/2 ripe avocado

1 egg

Salt and pepper to taste

Red pepper flakes (optional)

DIRECTIONS

1. Toast the bread to your liking.

2. Mash the avocado and spread it on the toast.

3. Fry the egg to your preference and place it on top of the avocado.

4. Season with salt, pepper, and red pepper flakes.

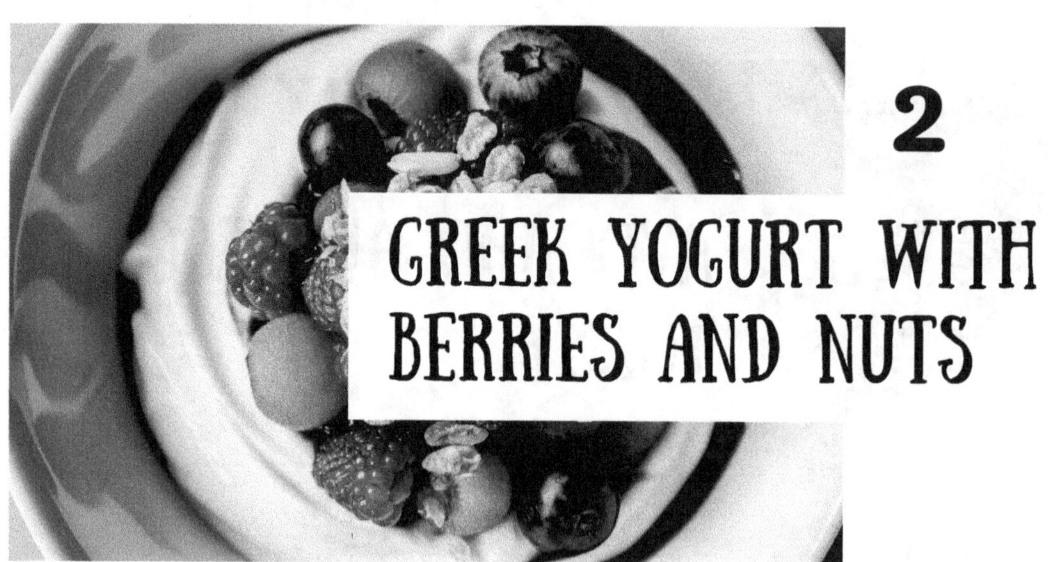

SERVINGS: 1   PREPPING TIME: 5 MIN

INGREDIENTS

1 cup Greek
yogurt
1/2 cup mixed
berries
1/4 cup mixed
nuts, chopped
1 tablespoon
honey

DIRECTIONS

- In a bowl, combine Greek yogurt and honey.
- Top with mixed berries and nuts before serving.

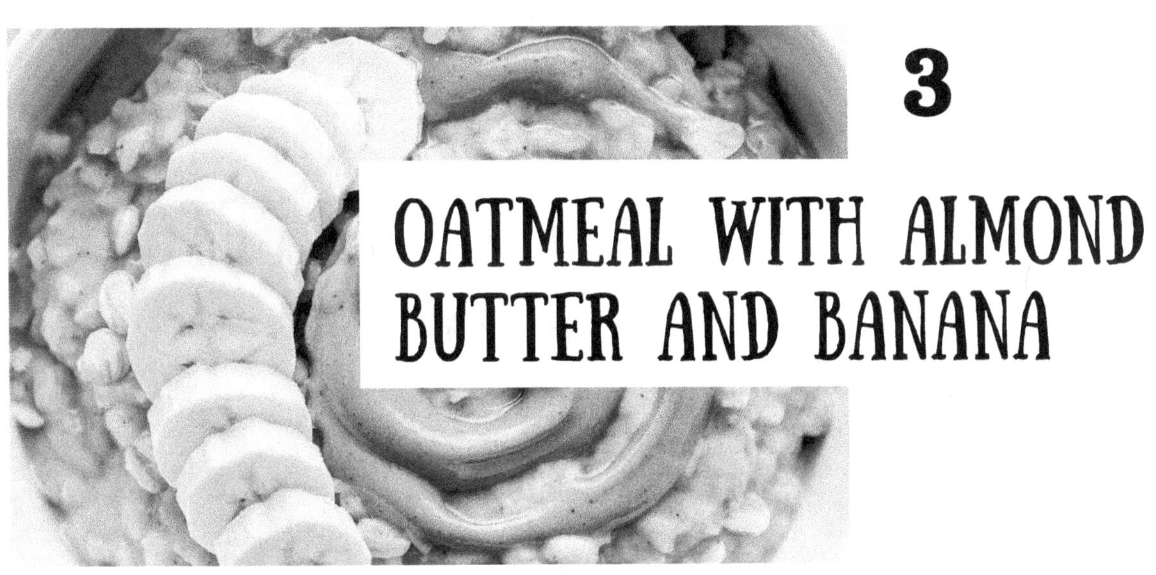

OATMEAL WITH ALMOND BUTTER AND BANANA

SERVINGS: 1   PREPPING TIME: 10 MIN

INGREDIENTS

1/2 cup rolled oats

1 cup almond milk

1 banana, sliced

1 tablespoon almond butter

Cinnamon to taste

DIRECTIONS

- Cook oats with almond milk according to package instructions.
- Stir in almond butter and top with banana slices and cinnamon.

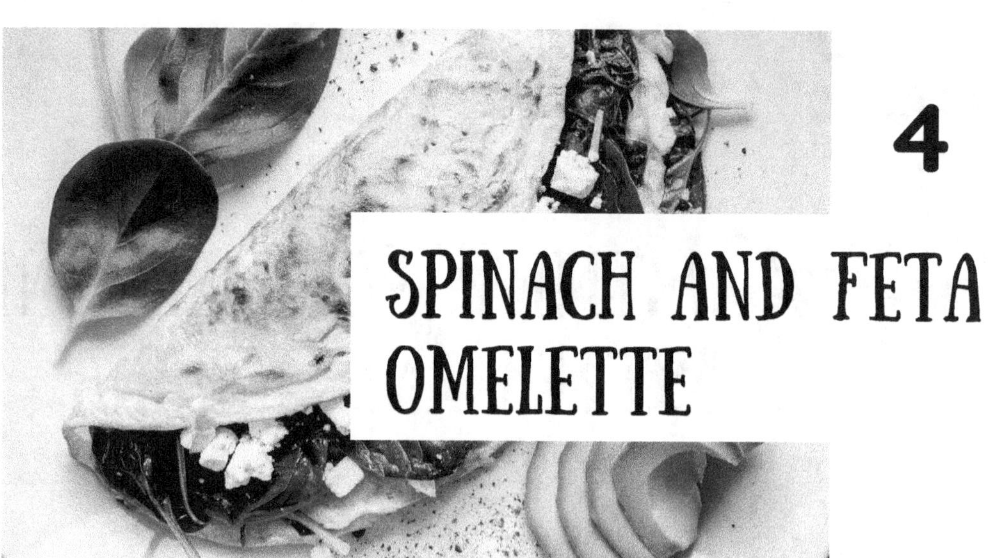

SPINACH AND FETA OMELETTE

4

SERVINGS: 1

PREPPING TIME: 15 MIN

INGREDIENTS

2 eggs

1 cup spinach, chopped

1/4 cup feta cheese, crumbled

Salt and pepper to taste

1 teaspoon olive oil

DIRECTIONS

- Beat the eggs with salt and pepper.
- Heat olive oil in a pan, sauté spinach until wilted.
- Pour eggs over spinach and sprinkle feta on top.
- Cook until eggs are set, fold omelette in half, and serve.

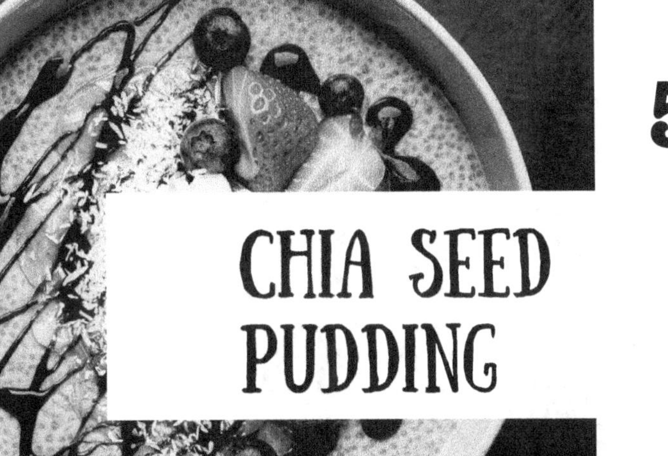

SERVINGS: 1   PREPPING TIME: 5 MIN

INGREDIENTS

3 tablespoons chia seeds

1 cup almond milk

1 tablespoon maple syrup

1/2 teaspoon vanilla extract

Fresh fruit for topping

DIRECTIONS

- Mix chia seeds, almond milk, maple syrup, and vanilla in a bowl.
- Refrigerate overnight until it thickens.
- Top with fresh fruit before serving.

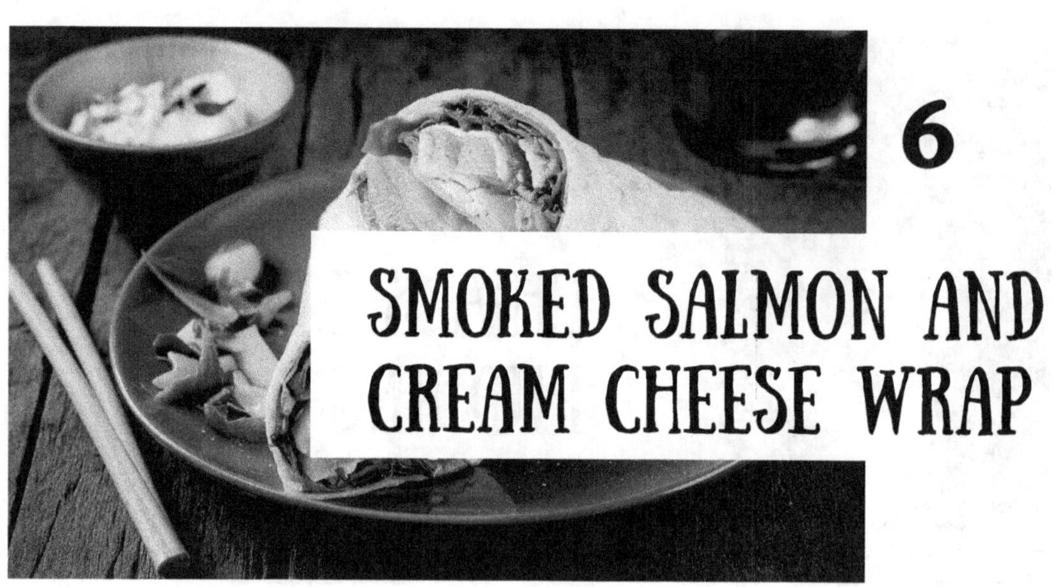

SERVINGS: 1

PREPPING TIME: 5 MIN

INGREDIENTS

1 whole-grain
wrap
2 tablespoons
cream cheese
2 ounces smoked
salmon
1/4 red onion,
thinly sliced
1 tablespoon
capers

DIRECTIONS

- Spread cream cheese on the wrap.
- Add smoked salmon, red onion, and capers.
- Roll up the wrap and slice in half to serve.

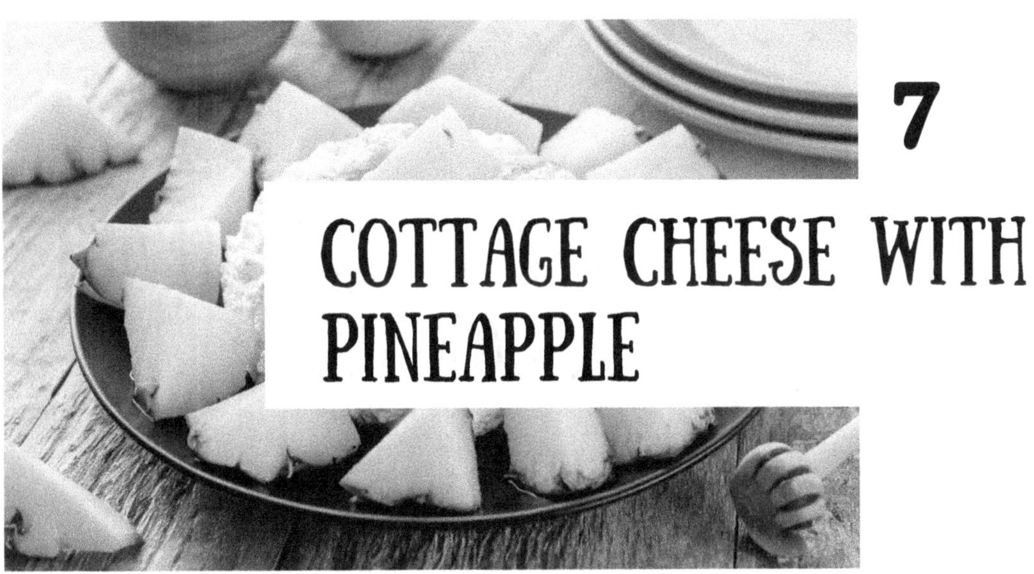

SERVINGS: 1

PREPPING TIME: 5 MIN

INGREDIENTS

1 cup cottage cheese

1/2 cup pineapple chunks

DIRECTIONS

- Simply combine cottage cheese and pineapple chunks in a bowl and enjoy.

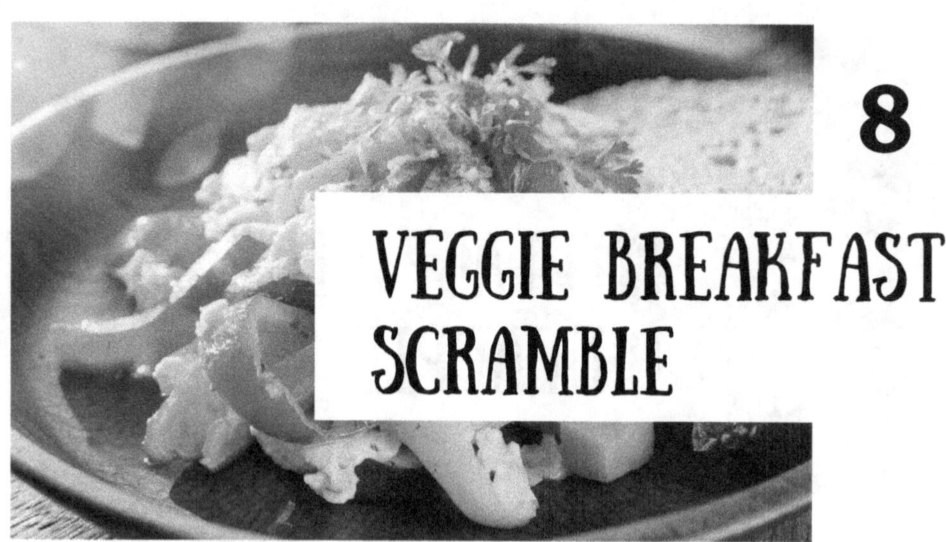

SERVINGS: 1   PREPPING TIME: 15 MIN

INGREDIENTS

2 eggs

1/2 cup bell peppers, diced

1/4 cup onions, diced

1/4 cup tomatoes, diced

1/4 cup shredded cheese

-Salt and pepper to taste

1 teaspoon olive oil

DIRECTIONS

- Heat olive oil in a pan and sauté bell peppers and onions until soft.

- Add beaten eggs, tomatoes, and cook until scrambled.

- Sprinkle cheese on top, season with salt and pepper, and serve.

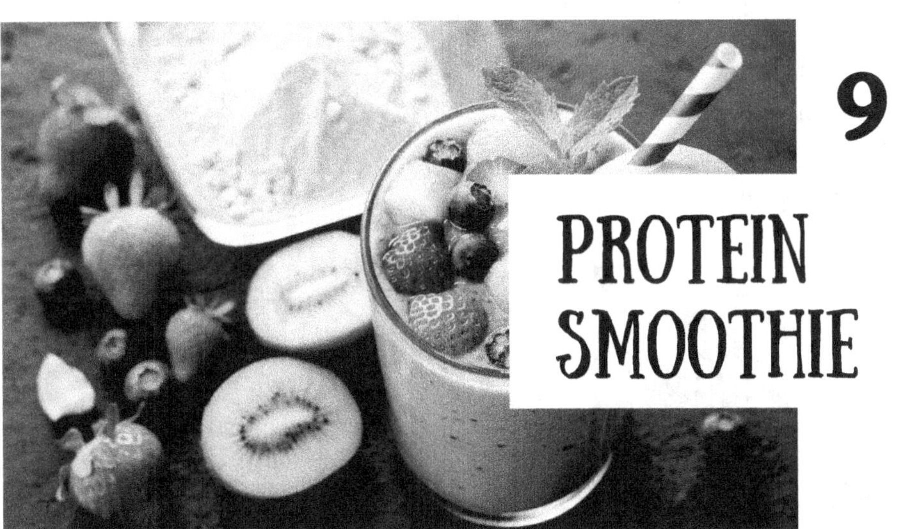

SERVINGS: 1   PREPPING TIME: 5 MIN

INGREDIENTS

1 scoop protein powder

1 cup almond milk

1/2 banana

1/2 cup frozen berries

1 tablespoon flaxseeds

DIRECTIONS

- Blend all ingredients until smooth and serve immediately.

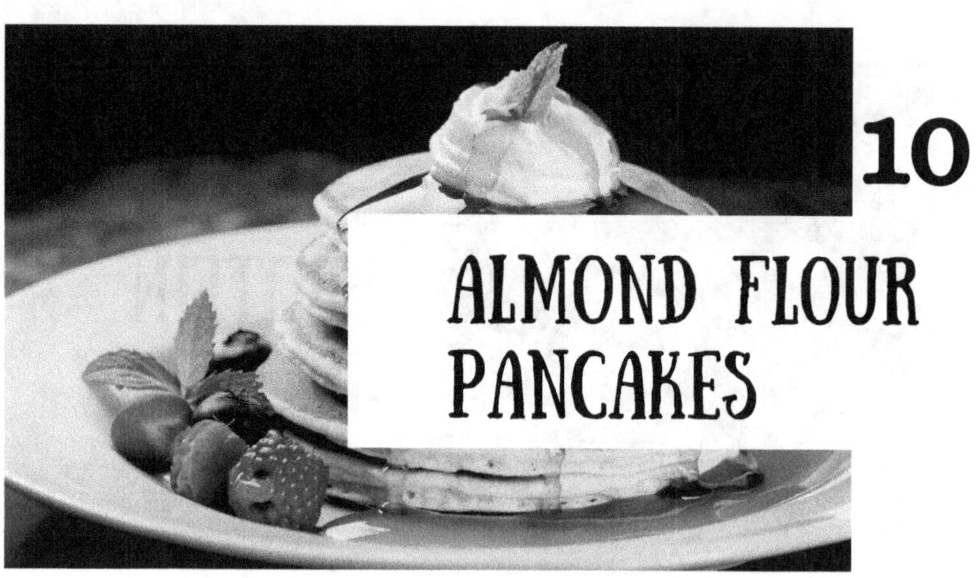

ALMOND FLOUR PANCAKES

10

SERVINGS: 2   PREPPING TIME: 20 MIN

INGREDIENTS

1 cup almond flour

2 eggs

1/3 cup almond milk

1 tablespoon maple syrup

1 teaspoon baking powder

Pinch of salt

Butter or oil for cooking

DIRECTIONS

- Mix almond flour, eggs, almond milk, maple syrup, baking powder, and salt in a bowl.
- Heat butter or oil in a pan and pour batter to form pancakes.
- Cook until bubbles form, flip, and cook the other side.
- Serve with your favorite low-calorie syrup or fresh berries.

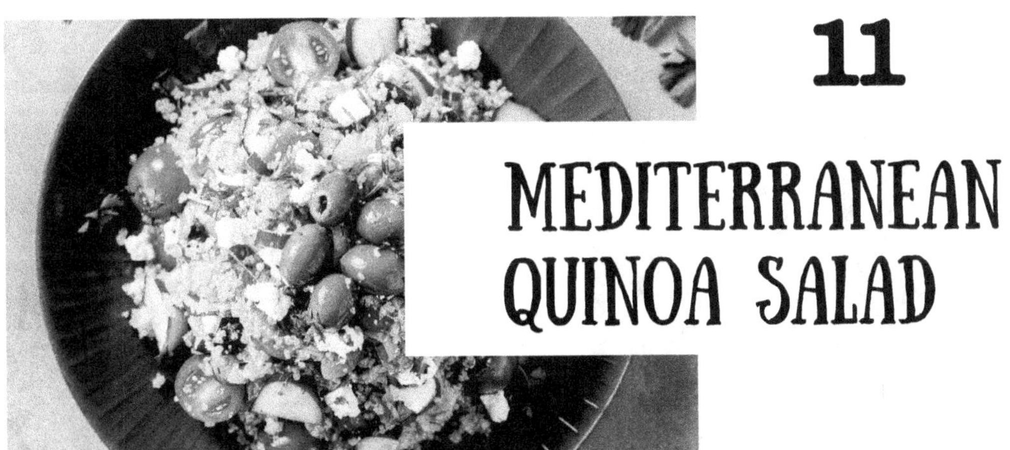

11

MEDITERRANEAN QUINOA SALAD

SERVINGS: 2   PREPPING TIME: 20 MIN

INGREDIENTS

1 cup cooked quinoa

1/2 cup cherry tomatoes, halved

1/2 cup cucumber, diced

1/4 cup red onion, finely chopped

1/4 cup feta cheese, crumbled

1/4 cup Kalamata olives, pitted and halved

2 tablespoons olive oil

1 tablespoon lemon juice

Salt and pepper to taste

DIRECTIONS

- In a large bowl, combine quinoa, tomatoes, cucumber, onion, feta, and olives.

- Drizzle with olive oil and lemon juice, then season with salt and pepper.

- Toss everything together and serve chilled or at room temperature.

57

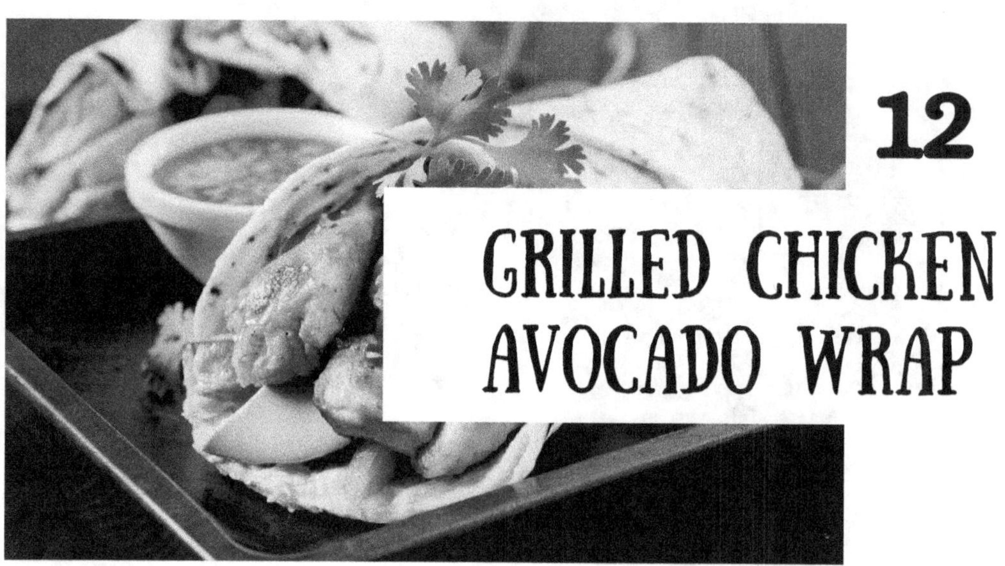

SERVINGS: 1   PREPPING TIME: 15 MIN

INGREDIENTS

1 whole-grain wrap

1 grilled chicken breast, sliced

1/2 ripe avocado, sliced

1/2 cup mixed greens

2 tablespoons Greek yogurt

Salt and pepper to taste

DIRECTIONS

- Lay the wrap flat and spread Greek yogurt over it.
- Add the chicken, avocado slices, and mixed greens.
- Season with salt and pepper, roll up the wrap tightly, and cut in half.

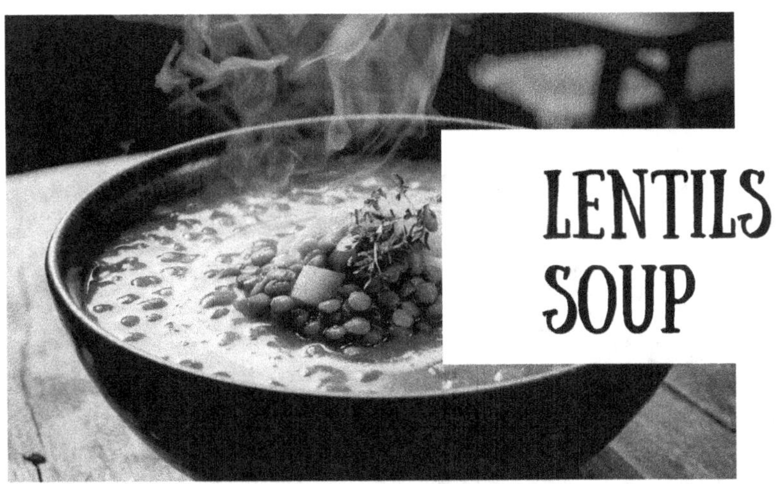

13

LENTILS SOUP

SERVINGS: 4 — PREPPING TIME: 45 MIN

INGREDIENTS

1 cup lentils, rinsed

1 onion, diced

2 carrots, diced

2 celery stalks, diced

2 garlic cloves, minced

1 can diced tomatoes

4 cups vegetable broth

1 teaspoon cumin

Salt and pepper to taste

1 tablespoon olive oil

DIRECTIONS

- Heat olive oil in a large pot over medium heat.
- Add onion, carrots, celery, and garlic. Cook until softened.
- Stir in lentils, tomatoes, broth, and cumin.
- Bring to a boil, then reduce heat and simmer until lentils are tender.
- Season with salt and pepper, and serve hot.

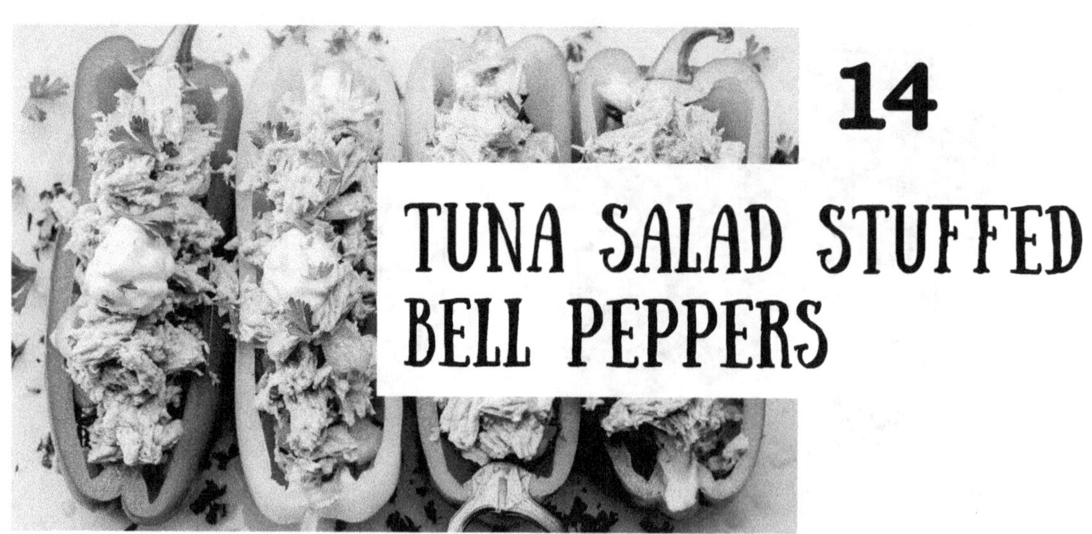

SERVINGS: 2	PREPPING TIME: 15 MIN

INGREDIENTS

2 bell peppers, halved
and seeded

1 can tuna, drained

1/4 cup mayonnaise

1/4 cup celery, diced

1 tablespoon red onion,
minced

1 tablespoon fresh
parsley, chopped

Salt and pepper to taste

DIRECTIONS

- In a bowl, mix together tuna, mayonnaise, celery, onion, and parsley.
- Season with salt and pepper.
- Spoon the tuna mixture into the bell pepper halves and serve.

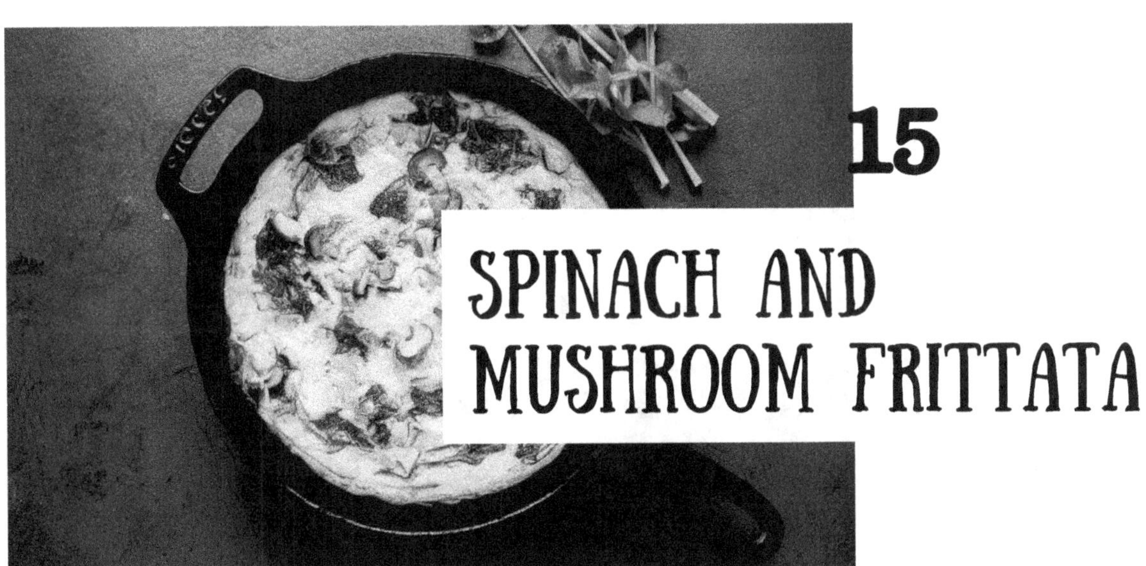

15

SPINACH AND MUSHROOM FRITTATA

INGREDIENTS

6 eggs

2 cups spinach, chopped

1 cup mushrooms, sliced

1/2 cup cheese, grated

Salt and pepper to taste

1 tablespoon olive oil

DIRECTIONS

- Preheat oven to 375°F (190°C).
- In a skillet, heat olive oil over medium heat. Sauté mushrooms until browned.
- Add spinach and cook until wilted.
- Beat eggs with salt and pepper, pour over vegetables in the skillet.
- Sprinkle cheese on top and transfer skillet to oven.
- Bake until eggs are set, about 15-20 minutes.

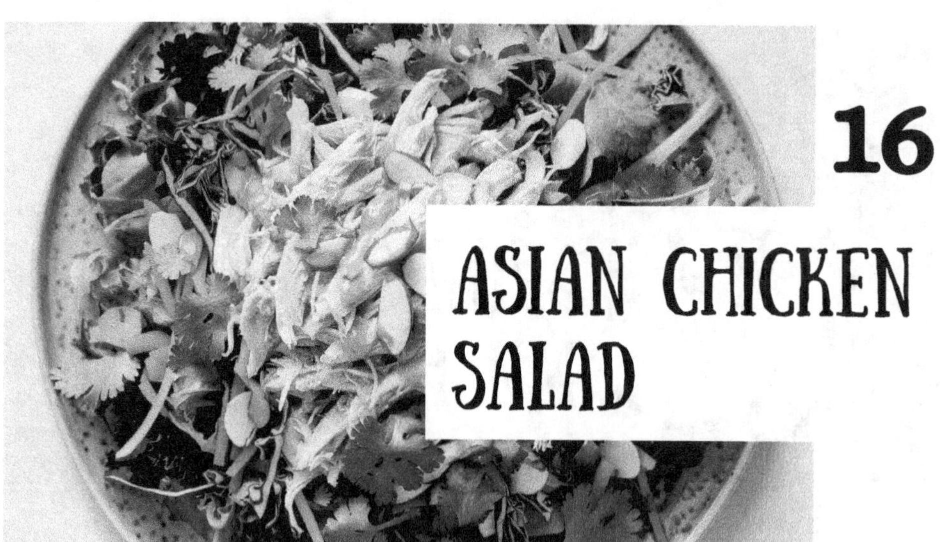

| SERVINGS: 2 | PREPPING TIME: 20 MIN |

INGREDIENTS

2 cups cooked chicken, shredded

4 cups mixed greens

1/2 cup red cabbage, shredded

1/2 cup carrots, julienned

1/4 cup cilantro, chopped

1/4 cup almonds, sliced

2 tablespoons sesame oil

1 tablespoon soy sauce

1 tablespoon rice vinegar

1 teaspoon honey

1 teaspoon ginger, grated

DIRECTIONS

- In a large bowl, combine chicken, greens, cabbage, carrots, and cilantro.

- In a small bowl, whisk together sesame oil, soy sauce, vinegar, honey, and ginger.

- Pour dressing over salad, toss to coat, and sprinkle with almonds.

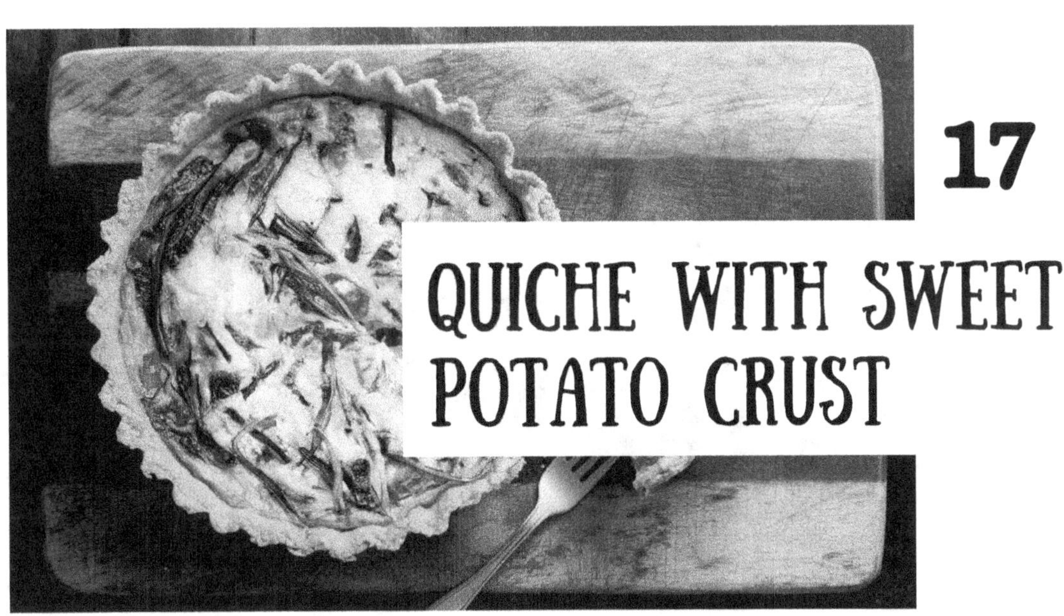

17

QUICHE WITH SWEET POTATO CRUST

SERVINGS: 4   PREPPING TIME: 1 HOUR

INGREDIENTS

large sweet potato, thinly sliced

6 eggs

1/2 cup milk

1 cup spinach, chopped

1/2 cup cheese, grated

Salt and pepper to taste

1 tablespoon olive oil

DIRECTIONS

- Preheat oven to 375°F (190°C).
- Grease a pie dish with olive oil and layer sweet potato slices to form a crust.
- Bake for 20 minutes until potatoes are slightly tender.
- Whisk together eggs, milk, salt, and pepper.
- Add spinach and cheese to the egg mixture, then pour into the sweet potato crust.
- Bake for 30-35 minutes until the quiche is set.

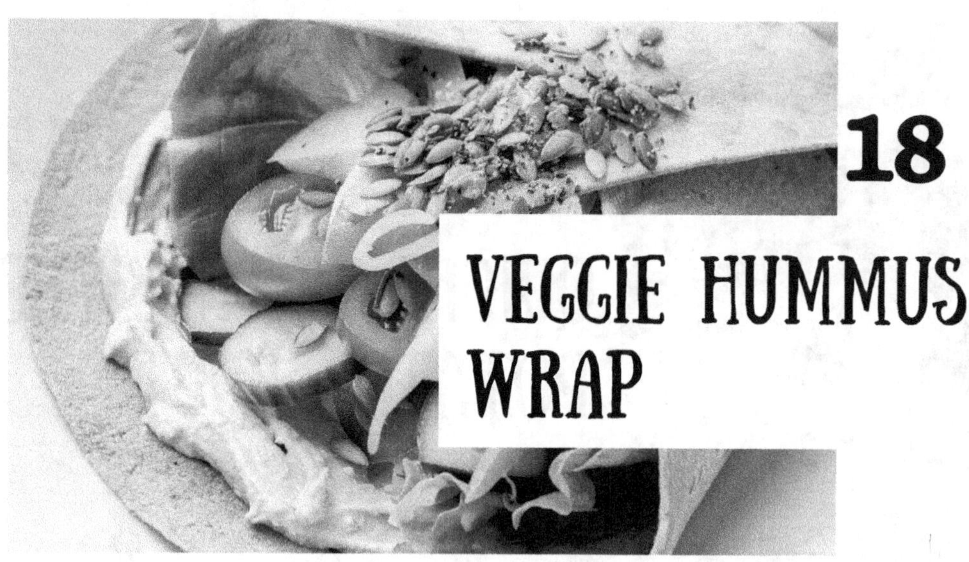

| SERVINGS: 1 | PREPPING TIME: 10 MINS |

INGREDIENTS

1 whole-grain wrap

3 tablespoons hummus

1/2 cup mixed greens

1/4 cup cucumber,

sliced

1/4 cup bell pepper,

sliced

1/4 cup carrot, shredded

1/4 avocado, sliced

DIRECTIONS

- Spread hummus on the wrap.
- Layer greens, cucumber, bell pepper, carrot, and avocado.
- Roll up the wrap tightly and cut in half

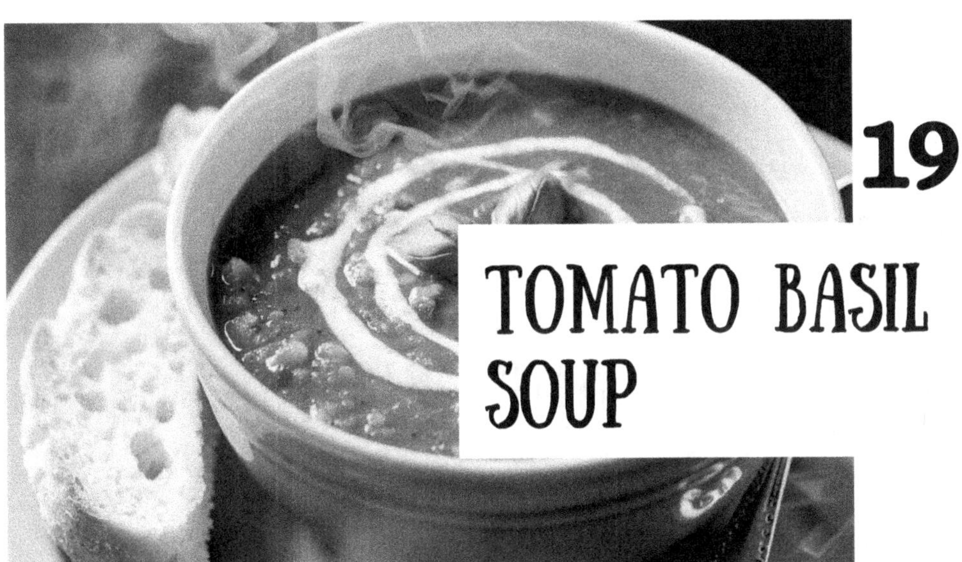

TOMATO BASIL SOUP

19

INGREDIENTS

1 can whole peeled tomatoes

1 onion, diced

2 garlic cloves, minced

2 cups vegetable broth

1/4 cup fresh basil, chopped

Salt and pepper to taste

1 tablespoon olive oil

DIRECTIONS

- Heat olive oil in a pot over medium heat.
- Add onion and garlic, cook until softened.
- Add tomatoes and broth, bring to a simmer.
- Use an immersion blender to puree the soup until smooth.
- Stir in basil, season with salt and pepper, and serve.

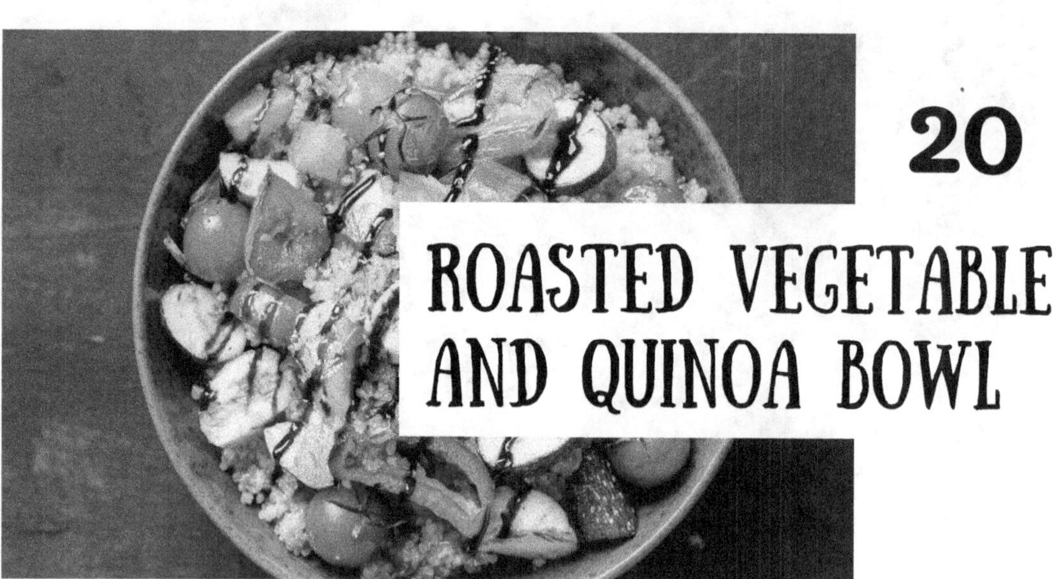

20

ROASTED VEGETABLE AND QUINOA BOWL

SERVINGS: 2   PREPPING TIME: 40 MINS

INGREDIENTS

1 cup quinoa, cooked

1 zucchini, sliced

1 bell pepper, sliced

1/2 red onion, sliced

1/2 cup cherry

tomatoes

1/4 cup feta cheese,

crumbled

2 tablespoons olive oil

Salt and pepper to taste

DIRECTIONS

- Preheat oven to 400°F (200°C).
- Toss zucchini, bell pepper, onion, and tomatoes with olive oil, salt, and pepper.
- Roast vegetables for 25-30 minutes until tender.
- Divide quinoa between bowls, top with roasted vegetables and feta cheese.

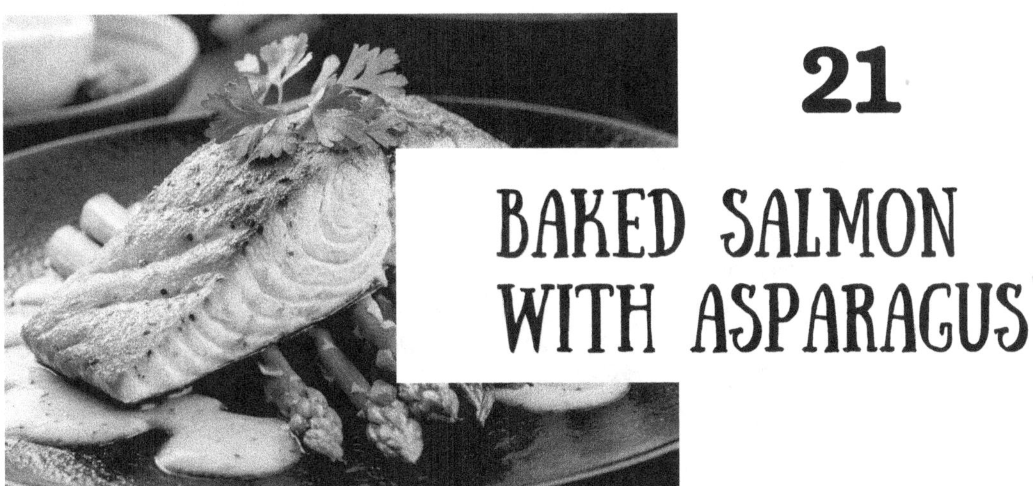

21
BAKED SALMON
WITH ASPARAGUS

SERVINGS: 2   PREPPING TIME: 25 MIN

INGREDIENTS

2 salmon fillets
1 bunch asparagus,
trimmed
2 tablespoons olive oil
1 lemon, sliced
Salt and pepper to taste

DIRECTIONS

- Preheat oven to 400°F (200°C).
- Place salmon and asparagus on a baking sheet.
- Drizzle with olive oil and season with salt and pepper.
- Top with lemon slices and bake for 15-20 minutes.

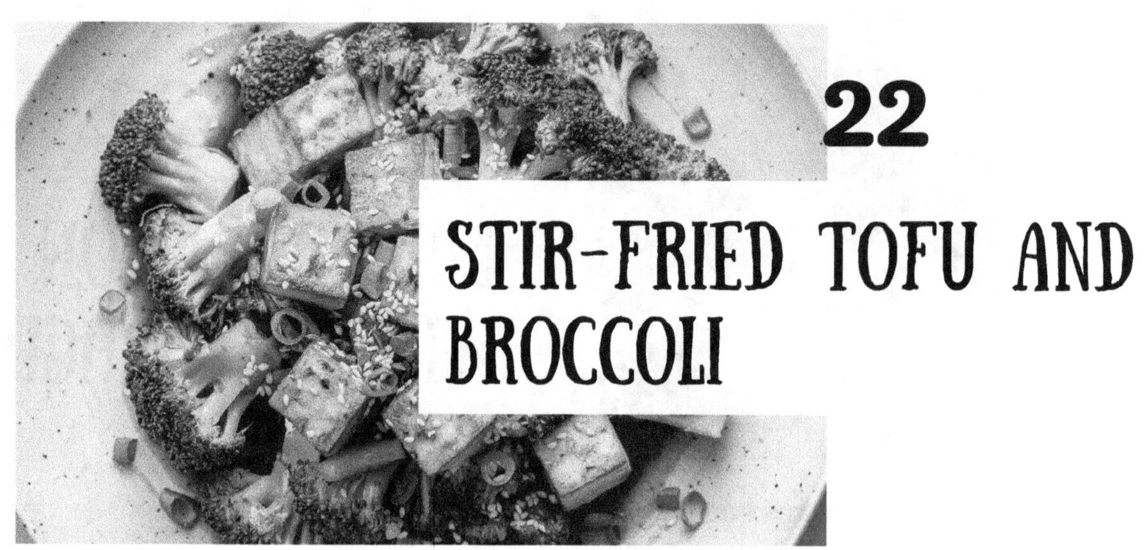

22

STIR-FRIED TOFU AND BROCCOLI

SERVINGS: 2   PREPPING TIME: 20 MINS

INGREDIENTS

1 block firm tofu, cubed

2 cups broccoli florets

1 tablespoon soy sauce

1 tablespoon sesame oil

1 garlic clove, minced

1 teaspoon ginger, grated

DIRECTIONS

- Heat sesame oil in a pan over medium heat.
- Add tofu and cook until golden brown.
- Add broccoli, garlic, and ginger. Stir-fry until broccoli is tender-crisp.
- Drizzle with soy sauce and serve.

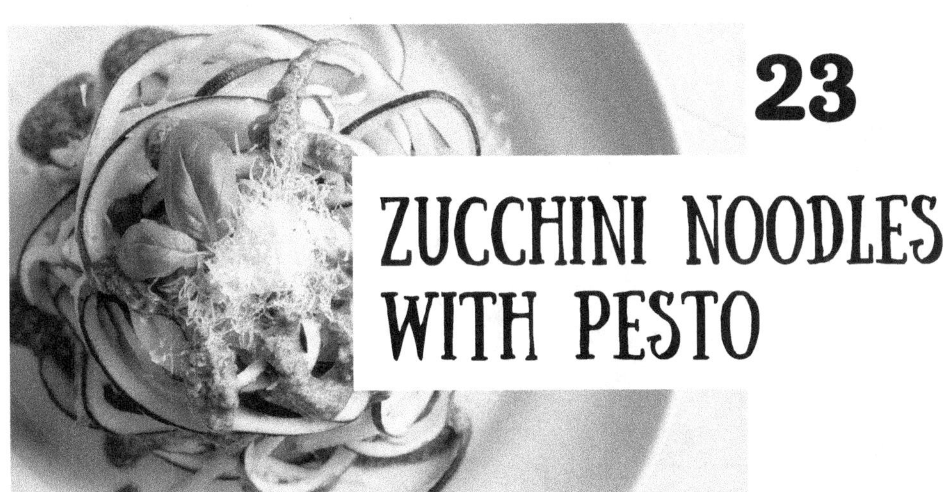

23

ZUCCHINI NOODLES WITH PESTO

INGREDIENTS

2 zucchinis, spiralized

1/4 cup pesto sauce

1/4 cup cherry tomatoes, halved

1/4 cup parmesan cheese, grated

DIRECTIONS

- In a pan, cook spiralized zucchini for 2-3 minutes.
- Remove from heat and mix in pesto sauce.
- Top with cherry tomatoes and parmesan cheese before serving.

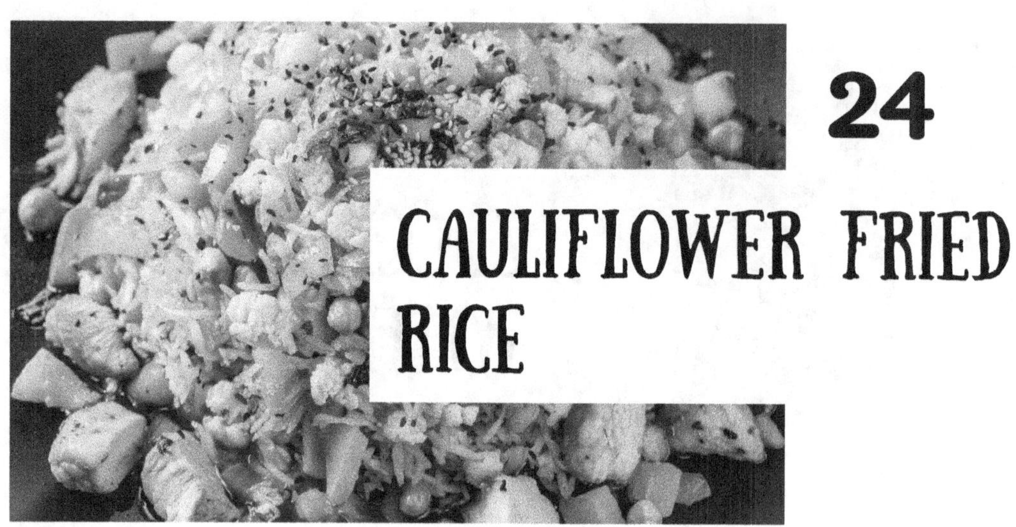

24

CAULIFLOWER FRIED RICE

INGREDIENTS

1 head cauliflower, riced

1/2 cup peas and carrots, frozen

2 eggs, beaten

2 tablespoons soy sauce

1 tablespoon sesame oil

1 green onion, chopped

DIRECTIONS

- Heat sesame oil in a pan over medium heat.
- Add cauliflower rice and frozen peas and carrots. Cook for 5-7 minutes.
- Push the mixture to one side of the pan, pour in eggs, and scramble.
- Stir everything together, add soy sauce, and garnish with green onions.

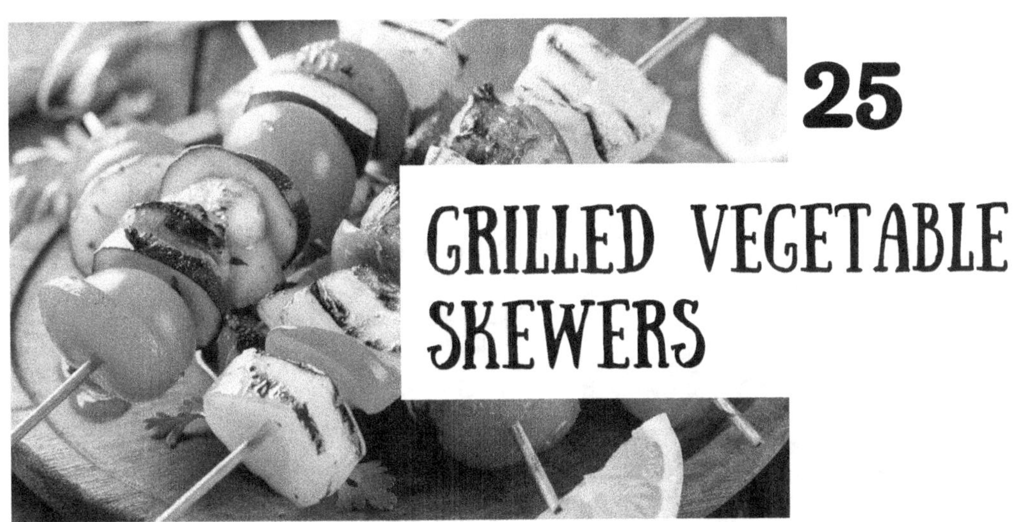

25

GRILLED VEGETABLE SKEWERS

INGREDIENTS

1 zucchini, cut into chunks

1 bell pepper, cut into chunks

1 red onion, cut into chunks

1 cup cherry tomatoes

2 tablespoons olive oil

1 tablespoon balsamic vinegar

Salt and pepper to taste

DIRECTIONS

- Thread vegetables onto skewers.
- Whisk together olive oil, balsamic vinegar, salt, and pepper.
- Brush the marinade over the skewers and let sit for at least 30 minutes.
- Grill over medium heat until vegetables are tender and slightly charred.

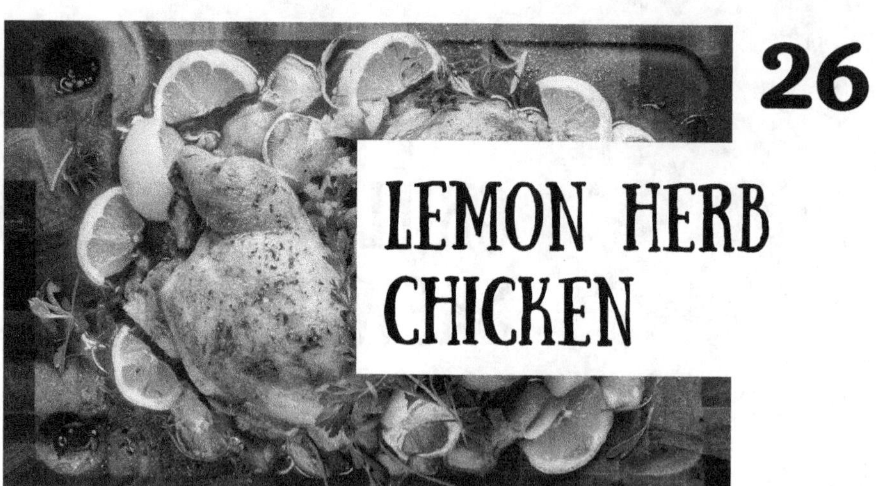

SERVINGS: 2   PREPPING TIME: 40 MINS

INGREDIENTS

2 chicken breasts

2 tablespoons olive oil

1 lemon, juiced and
zested

1 tablespoon fresh
herbs (thyme, rosemary,
parsley), chopped

Salt and pepper to taste

DIRECTIONS

- Preheat oven to 375°F (190°C).
- 2. In a bowl, mix olive oil, lemon juice and zest, herbs, salt, and pepper.
- 3. Coat chicken breasts with the mixture and bake for 25-30 minutes.

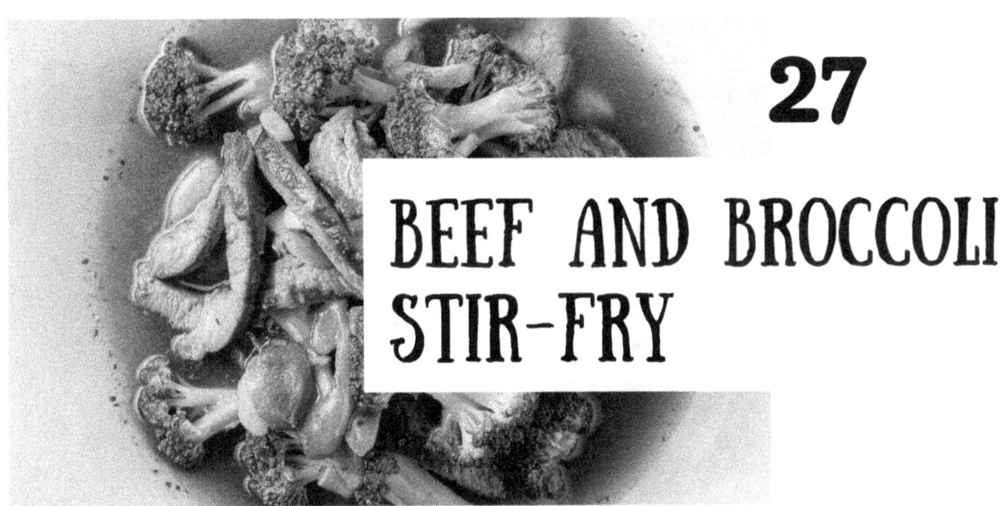

SERVINGS: 2   PREPPING TIME: 20 MINS

INGREDIENTS

1/2 pound beef, thinly sliced

2 cups broccoli florets

1 tablespoon soy sauce

1 tablespoon oyster sauce

1 teaspoon cornstarch

1 tablespoon vegetable oil

DIRECTIONS

- In a bowl, mix soy sauce, oyster sauce, and cornstarch with a little water.
- Heat oil in a pan and cook beef until browned.
- Add broccoli and the sauce mixture. Cook until the sauce thickens.

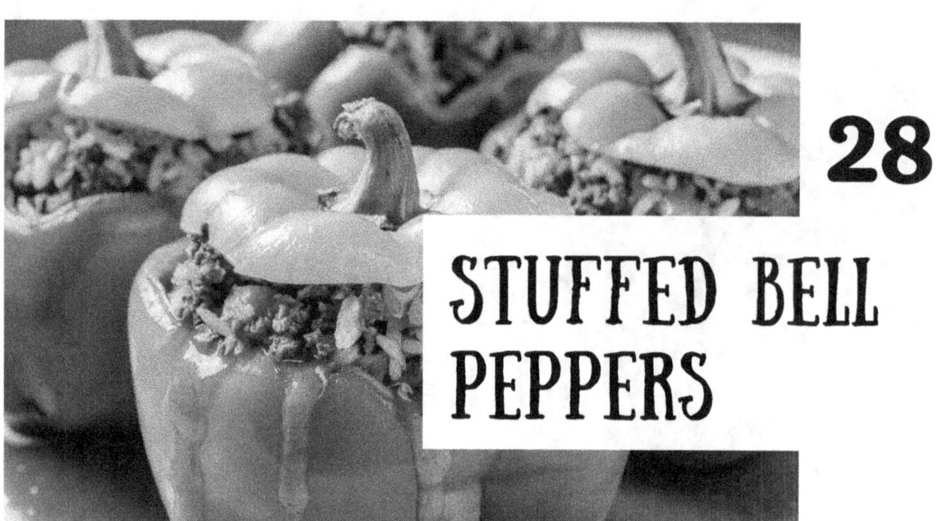

28
STUFFED BELL PEPPERS

SERVINGS: 4   PREPPING TIME: 1 HOUR

INGREDIENTS

4 bell peppers, tops removed and seeded

1/2 pound ground turkey

1 cup cooked quinoa

1 can diced tomatoes

1/2 onion, diced

1 garlic clove, minced

1 teaspoon cumin

1/2 cup cheese, shredded

Salt and pepper to taste

1 tablespoon olive oil

DIRECTIONS

- Preheat oven to 350°F (175°C).
- In a pan, heat olive oil and cook onion and garlic until soft.
- Add ground turkey, cook until browned.
- Stir in quinoa, tomatoes, cumin, salt, and pepper.
- Stuff the mixture into bell peppers, top with cheese.
- Bake for 30 minutes until peppers are tender.

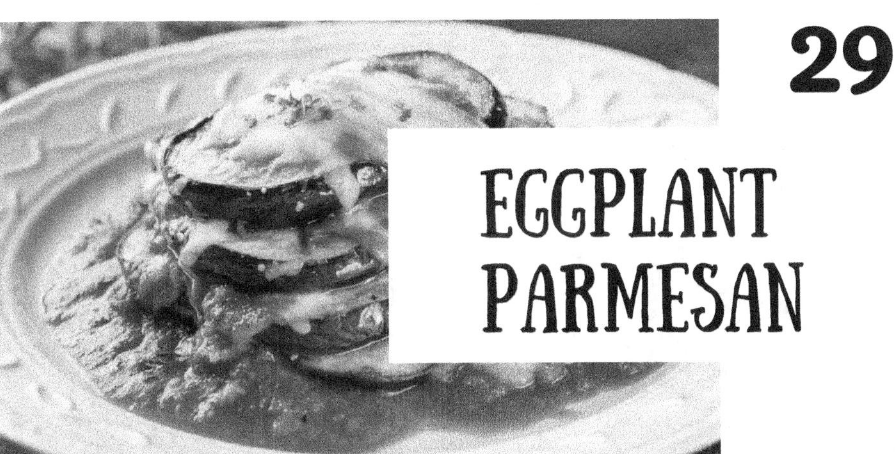

29

EGGPLANT PARMESAN

INGREDIENTS

large eggplant, sliced
into rounds

2 cups marinara sauce

1 cup mozzarella
cheese, shredded

1/2 cup parmesan
cheese, grated

1/4 cup basil leaves,
chopped

Salt and pepper to taste

Olive oil for cooking

DIRECTIONS

- Preheat oven to 375°F (190°C).
- Season eggplant slices with salt and pepper.
- In a skillet, cook eggplant in olive oil until browned on both sides.
- In a baking dish, layer marinara sauce, eggplant, mozzarella, and parmesan.
- Repeat layers and finish with cheese on top.
- Bake for 25-30 minutes until cheese is bubbly and golden.

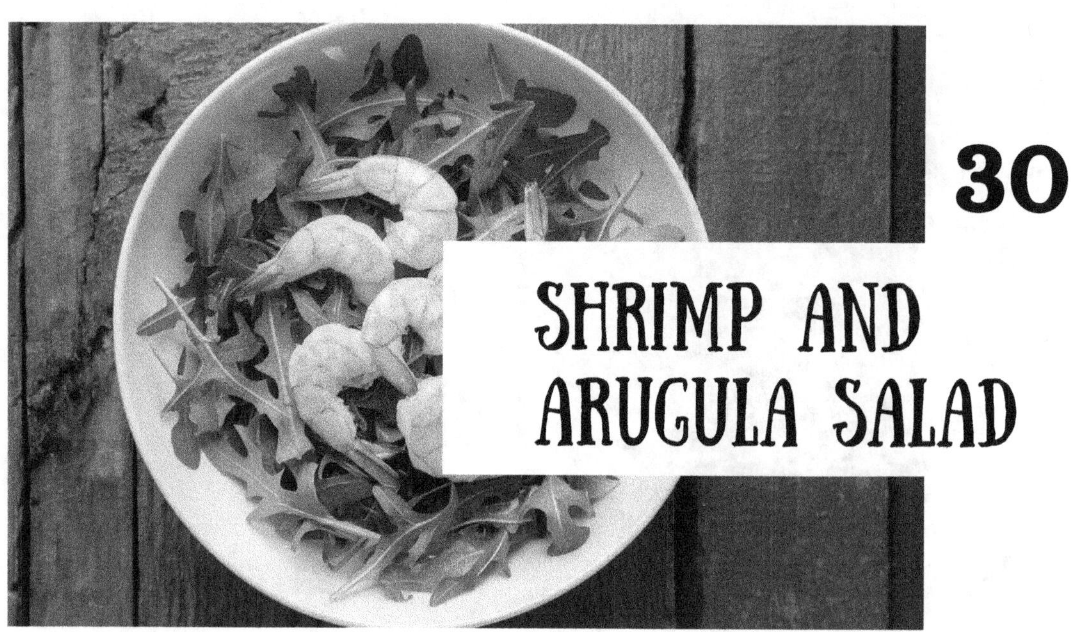

30

SHRIMP AND ARUGULA SALAD

INGREDIENTS

1/2 pound shrimp, peeled and
deveined

4 cups arugula

1/2 avocado, sliced

1/4 cup cherry tomatoes,
halved

1/4 cup cucumber, sliced

2 tablespoons olive oil

1 tablespoon lemon juice

Salt and pepper to taste

DIRECTIONS

- Preheat oven to 375°F (190°C).
- Season eggplant slices with salt and pepper.
- In a skillet, cook eggplant in olive oil until browned on both sides.
- In a baking dish, layer marinara sauce, eggplant, mozzarella, and parmesan.
- Repeat layers and finish with cheese on top.
- Bake for 25-30 minutes until cheese is bubbly and golden.

OVERCOMING CHALLENGES

DEALING WITH SOCIAL SITUATIONS

Meals are a common focal point of social gatherings, so planning beforehand is crucial. It's crucial to realise that you may still engage and socialise with others even if you eat outside of your fasting time.

Explaining Your IF Technique
- Be Open: To help friends and family understand your eating routine, feel free to discuss your IF practice with them.
- Provide Options: Encourage gatherings for non-food-related events like walks, reading clubs, or cultural gatherings.

Getting Ready
- Modify Your Schedule: If at all possible, change the window during which you fast to coincide with the event.
- Eat Beforehand: Eat a healthy supper in order to reduce your temptation to eat outside of your designated eating window.

During the Event
- Remain Hydrated: To stay hydrated and control hunger, always have a glass of water on hand.
- Situational Attention: Shift the emphasis from eating to conversing and socialising with others.
- Politely Decline: Saying "I've already eaten" or "I'm not hungry right now" is sufficient when offered food.

Conscious Engagement
- Enjoy Non-Food Aspects: Take in the décor, music, and atmosphere.

- If it's a potluck, Bring Your Own Dish: Provide a dish that is in line with your IF menu.
- Eat With Mindfulness: If you decide to eat, do so with awareness, enjoying every taste and being aware of your body's hunger signals.

How to Respond to Inquiries and Peer Pressure
- Prepare Responses: Be prepared with a couple answers in case someone asks you why you're not eating.
- Remain assured: Have faith in the decisions you make. You owe no one an explanation about your food choices.

It takes courage, communication, and planning to navigate social situations on an IF schedule. You can enjoy social gatherings without worrying that your fasting schedule is being jeopardised by using these techniques.

EMOTIONAL EATING AND FASTING

Emotional eating is the practice of eating to satisfy emotions rather than hunger. It is crucial to differentiate between eating for sustenance and eating motivated by feelings like boredom, tension, or melancholy.

Determining Firearms
- Maintain a Food Journal: Monitor your consumption patterns and record your feelings when you grab for food.
- Identify Patterns: Keep an eye out for reoccurring events or emotions that lead you to eat beyond the window of fasting.

Creating Coping Mechanisms
- Mindfulness Techniques: Use mindfulness to remain in the present moment and identify emotional cues.

- Stress Management: Take part in stress-relieving exercises, such as yoga, meditation, or light exercise.
- Seek Support: Instead of turning to food, discuss your feelings with friends, family, or a professional.

Healthy Substitutes
- Discover New Interests: Engage in hands-on and mental hobbies like knitting, painting, or gardening.
- Schedule Entertaining Non-Food Activities: Plan enjoyable activities for yourself that don't require food.

At Times of Fasting
- Remain Hydrated: To help control cravings, sip on water or herbal tea.
- Distract Yourself: Take a walk or curl up with a nice book to help divert your attention if you're feeling tempted to eat because of feelings.

Changing the Way You View Food
- Food as Nourishment: Change your mindset so that you see food as your body's sustenance rather than as a crutch for your emotions.
- Celebrate Non-Scale Victories: Pay attention to the advantages of IF that go beyond mere weight loss.

Controlling one's emotional eating is essential to a successful

ADJUSTMENTS YOUR PLAN AS YOUR AGE

Women's bodies and lives alter even more as they age into their 60s and beyond. Plans for intermittent fasting (IF) may need to be modified to account for these modifications.

Your metabolism naturally decreases with age. This could have an impact on how your body reacts to fasting and necessitate modifying your IF schedule or calorie intake.

Modifying the Window for Fasting
- Listen to Your Body: During times of fasting, be mindful of your body's feelings. If you feel lethargic, you might need to reduce the length of your fasting period.
- Remain Adaptable: Be open to adjusting your fasting schedule in light of your present state of health and level of exercise.

Changing Food Requirement
- Nutrient Density: Give special attention to foods high in nutrients that promote bone health, muscle upkeep, and mental clarity.
- Hydration: Since older persons are more prone to dehydration, make hydration a priority.

Including Physical Activity
- Low-Impact Activities: Incorporate joint-friendly workouts such as yoga, swimming, and walking.
- Strength Training: To preserve bone density and muscular mass, keep up your modest strength training.

Keeping an Eye on Health Markers
- Regular Check-Ups: Attend your doctor's appointments on time to keep an eye on vital signs including blood pressure, cholesterol, and sugar levels.
- Consult Medical Professionals: Make sure your IF plan supports your medical needs by collaborating with your healthcare team.

Emotional and Social Welfare
- Social Engagement: Find methods to integrate IF without isolating yourself. Social ties are essential for mental well-being.

- Mental Health: Take care of your mental well-being and get help if you feel depressed or alone.

Finding balance and continuing to respect your body's demands are key to modifying your IF plan as you get older. You can continue to reap the benefits of intermittent fasting (IF) and sustain an active and healthy lifestyle well into your 60s and beyond with some careful tweaks.

It's vital to consider the significant insights and lessons that intermittent fasting brings as we turn the last pages of this trip to a conclusion. For women over sixty, this is a transforming experience that is in harmony with ageing and life's natural cycles, not just a change in food.

Beyond helping you reduce weight or speed up your metabolism, intermittent fasting can help you rediscover your body's natural ability to repair and regenerate. By comprehending the science of fasting and putting this guide's recommended behaviours into practice, you've given yourself the means to age gracefully and vibrantly.

Not only are the personal accounts, dietary recommendations, and recipe books helpful, but they also serve as stepping stones towards a sustainable way of living. They stand as an example of the strength that can be achieved through perseverance and the support of a group of like-minded people.

Keep in mind that the joy of living life to the fullest and the quality of life are the real indicators of success as you modify and refine your fasting plan. This is just the beginning of the trip; learning, developing, and thriving are continuous processes.

I hope this book stays with you always as you look forward to a healthy, happy, and wiser-than-you-age future. Cheers to a well-lived life, well-nourished body, and well-fulfilled spirit.

21 DAYS MEAL PLAN

NOTE:

- For the first week meal plan, numbers are written on each recipes, you can trace them to the recipes in the book that has that number for identification

- For the second and third week, there is no need to trace, the names are there already, just follow them and your intermittent fasting journey will be smooth

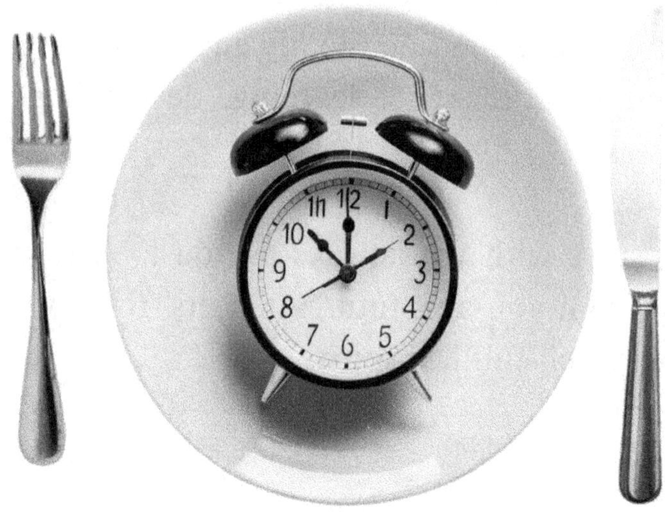

	Breakfast	Launch	Dinner
Sunday	3	19	21
Monday	2	18	22
Tuesday	4	17	23
Wednesday	5	16	24
Thursday	6	15	25
Friday	7	14	26
Saturday	10	13	27

	Breakfast	Launch	Dinner
Sunday	Chia seed pudding with fresh berries.	Spinach and feta stuffed chicken breast	Grilled eggplant and zucchini lasagna.
Monday	Greek yogurt with sliced almonds	Tuna salad with mixed leafy greens,	Roasted turkey breast with brussels sprouts
Tuesday	Scrambled eggs with spinach and mushrooms.	Lentil and vegetable stew with a slice of whole-grain bread	Baked cod with a side of steamed green beans and almonds.
Wednesday	Poached eggs on whole-grain toast with avocado.	Broccoli and cheddar soup with a side of apple slices.	Beef stir-fry with bell peppers, onions, and snap peas over wild rice.
Thursday	Cottage cheese with pineapple chunks and flaxseeds.	Turkey and avocado wrap with a side of carrot sticks.	Stir-fried tofu with mixed vegetables over brown rice.
Friday	Smoothie with spinach, avocado, protein powder, and almond milk.	Chickpea salad with cucumbers, tomatoes, and parsley.	Grilled salmon with a side of roasted cauliflower and a mixed greens salad.
Saturday	Quinoa salad with roasted beets, goat cheese, and walnuts.	Baked lemon garlic chicken with asparagus and quinoa.	Oatmeal with sliced banana and a sprinkle of cinnamon.

	Breakfast	Launch	Dinner
Sunday	Mixed berry parfait with layers of Greek yogurt and granola.	Caprese salad with fresh mozzarella, tomatoes, basil, and balsamic glaze.	Garlic shrimp stir-fry with a medley of colorful vegetables over brown rice.
Monday	Almond butter and banana on whole-grain toast.	Greek salad with olives, feta, cucumber, and a light olive oil dressing.	Lemon herb roasted chicken with a side of green beans and roasted potatoes.
Tuesday	Baked avocado egg boats with a sprinkle of cheddar cheese.	Spinach and goat cheese omelet with a side of sliced tomatoes.	Grilled mahi-mahi with mango salsa and a quinoa salad.
Wednesday	Protein smoothie with mixed berries, spinach, and almond butter	Chicken Caesar salad with romaine lettuce, parmesan, and whole-grain croutons.	Vegetarian chili with a variety of beans and vegetables.
Thursday	Avocado toast with cherry tomatoes and poached egg.	Quinoa and black bean salad with corn, red peppers, and cilantro.	Pork tenderloin with roasted brussels sprouts and a side salad.
Friday	Whole-grain pancakes with blueberries and a dollop of Greek yogurt.	Lentil soup with a side of mixed berries.	Baked tilapia with a side of steamed broccoli and sweet potato.
Saturday	Almond butter and banana on whole-grain toast.	Grilled shrimp over mixed greens with a lemon vinaigrette.	Roast chicken with Mediterranean vegetables and couscous.